I0475060

Toxic Health

Cover Picture: A rainbow around the Sun can be a sign of atmospheric pollution and it may be a health issue.

Contents

Introduction

Toxic Health takes a look at the modern human environment and investigates how it is impacting human health. Modern industrialized humans have adopted habits and lifestyles that did not exist even just a few years ago. Each change in lifestyle generally has a cost to pay in terms of health.

Many small changes in lifestyle can add up to large problems that are accumulating in the human mind and body and show up many years later. The modern human has adopted a lifestyle that for many comes to a crashing halt in middle age as problems such as depression, aches and pains, diabetes, high cholesterol, forgetfulness, and a loss of vitality become the norm. We are in a time like no other in human history and we are now seeing the onset of these symptoms much earlier in the human as many children are not developing correctly.

The Institute of Health Metrics and Evaluations, University of Washington, reported in 2011 that the American average life expectancy is now in decline. Ranked a lowly 38th in the world, with 1 in 8 women now getting breast cancer. In some parts of the USA the average life expectancy is just 66 years.

People have fooled themselves into thinking that by taking a cocktail of vitamin supplements and prescription pills that they will get better. The reality is that this behavior just covers up underlying problems that are getting worse. Modern society is now filled with people who have falsely pinned their hopes for the future on medications.

With approximately 50% of the USA population on prescription drugs and 10% on anti-depressants, it is clear that things are going seriously wrong with human health in the modern world.

A concerning development is that approximately 300,000 people in Sweden have registered as having Electromagnetic Hypersensitivity (EHS). EHS is caused by exposure to electrical, electronic and wireless products and Sweden is the only country that currently recognizes it as a health condition. This new epidemic in the population is predicted to keep on increasing as the use of technology gains momentum.

It does not have to be this way. After years of extensive research into human health, Toxic Health has discovered that most of these symptoms are a product of toxins that we willingly have introduced into our lifestyles and by removing them we may restore the vitality back into our lives. There is a large and extensive web of these toxins and we will look into them and identify potential health hazards.

Good health for your entire life is completely dependent on your lifestyle choices and the environments that you spend time in. Toxic Health will discuss the changes necessary to work towards a positively healthy life. Toxic Health demonstrates how to live to a good age with a healthy and painless life that is free of prescription drugs.

Diagrams and photographs are used to illustrate many of the concepts of the book. If you are reading this in black and white, descriptions of the pictures accompany them to explain the concepts. The contents of the book should be accessible to most people through the visual explanations of subjects discussed in the book.

This book is aimed at the general public, the medical profession and the engineering profession. Mathematics is avoided and the book presents the concepts of the various forms of health in a readable format to the general public. Important points are in bold font.

This book contains the very latest research on health and the human environment. It should be viewed as the current ideas and the contents are subject to review by the scientific community. The author and publisher accept no liability whatsoever for any of the contents and the book is published in the spirit of unrestricted access to the latest ideas and scientific theories in a changing world.

You should always consult with a licensed and certified medical professional on any aspects of health, sickness or disease.

"The way you think, the way you behave, the way you eat, can influence your life by 30 to 50 years."

Deepak Chopra

Basics

We know that the human cannot survive without air, water and food and these are classed as the nutrition of the human body. But if you think that is all you need to worry about, then you may eventually develop poor health. Human nutrition is far more extensive and we have a comprehensive list below:

- Air.
- Water.
- Food.
- Exercise.
- Body voltage.
- Smells.
- Temperature.
- Humidity.
- Light.
- Sleep.
- Radiation.
- Metals.
- Altitude.
- Sounds and Vibrations.
- Chemical Exposure.
- Society.

The above are all nutritional items that need to be correct in order for you to be well. It just takes some simple steps to ensure that you have an excellent chance of achieving a long and healthy life that is free of pain.

As we can see in the next table, the modern human is currently dying of three leading things:

- **Heart and circulation.**
- **Cancer.**
- **Brain issues.**

The following diagram shows the age where people start to die from these things. As can be seen, the rate of death starts significantly rising from 30 years of age onwards.

Research conducted for Toxic Health is indicating that these three leading causes of death are preventable and it just takes a lifestyle adjustment to significantly reduce the risk of succumbing to these ailments.

"Liberty is to the collective body, what health is to every individual body. Without health, no pleasure can be tasted by man; Without liberty, no happiness can be enjoyed by society."

Henry St. John

Top 15 Causes of Death in the U.S. (2007)

Rank	Ages 1–85+	Rank	Ages 1–85+	Rank	Ages 1–85+
1	Heart Disease 615,616	6	Alzheimer's Disease 74,629	11	Septicemia 34,543
2	Malignant Neoplasms 562,795	7	Diabetes Mellitus 71,373	12	Liver Disease 29,158
3	Cerebrovascular 135,814	8	Influenza and Pneumonia 52,492	13	Hypertension 23,963
4	Chronic Lower Respiratory Disease 127,875	9	Nephritis 46,304	14	Parkinson's Disease 20,056
5	Unintentional Injury 122,387	10	Suicide 34,592	15	Homicide 17,984

Data courtesy of CDC

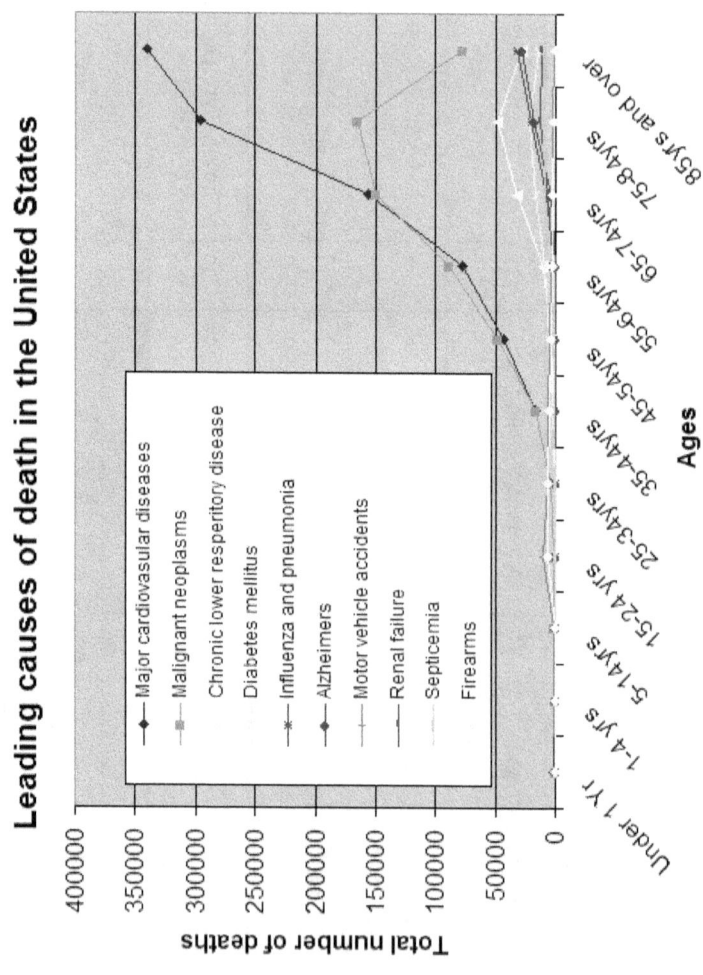

Leading causes of death in the United States

Air

Air quality is very important. Unfortunately, the industrialization of modern society has brought with it problems in air quality on a global scale. The air composition today has never existed in all of human history and it is getting worse every year. The addiction of using the air for dumping gases into by the modern human is having far reaching consequences for all life on the planet.

Indoor air can be made toxic by the use of household chemicals. Some seemingly innocent chemical products may have the ability to make you ill. Just leaving a bucket of household cleaner in the home for several days may fill the home with particles that you cannot sense. You will just notice that you are starting to get ill. It is important to use cleaning products only for short periods of time and in well ventilated spaces. Throw away any mixed products after you are done with cleaning.

Carbon monoxide poisoning can be an issue and it is odorless. This generally comes from sources of flames, such as gas heaters and fireplaces. Typically it comes from a blocked flue where the gasses come into the home instead of escaping to the outdoors. It can come from a garage if you have the car running too long in there. The symptoms to look for are:

- Headache.
- Dizziness.
- Nausea.
- Flu-like symptoms.
- Fatigue.
- Shortness of breath on exertion.
- Impaired judgment.

- Chest pain.
- Confusion.
- Depression.
- Hallucinations.
- Agitation.
- Vomiting.
- Abdominal pain.
- Drowsiness.
- Visual changes.
- Fainting.
- Seizure.
- Memory problems.
- Walking problems.

Air conditioners may have very good air quality in winter when they burn air to heat it. This draws fresh air into the home. They may have very poor air quality in the summertime when no air is drawn into the home due to cooling. ASHRAE (American Society of Heating, Refrigerating and Air Conditioning Engineers) recommends that 20 cubic feet per minute (CFM) of fresh air per person be drawn into a building for good air quality. You may need to install a fresh air vent in order to achieve this.

The top thing you can do to improve your indoor air quality is to ventilate the home to the outside air by opening the windows. Even if it is a hot or cold day, at least one window in your home should be opened slightly to allow air exchanges to take place.

So how can we gauge the progression of air pollution? The answer turns out to be relatively easy. Humans have been painting sunsets and moon-sets for hundreds of years in their artwork. Fortunately, much of this artwork has been kept in pristine condition and is available to view.

When reviewing the artwork of sunsets and moon-sets, we see that the orange and red colors appear to be a relatively modern phenomenon. Prior to this, they did not appear to be orange or red, they were relatively white.

Evidence of atmospheric pollution will be at its peak when the Sun or the Moon is near to the horizon. This is due to the radiation from these objects passing through the thickest part of the atmosphere. This is called "high air mass" in the scientific community. The radiation is subjected to the most atmospheric filtration at this time. Air mass is 1 when the Sun or Moon is at zenith and down at the horizon it is approximately 38. This means that the radiation receives 38 times more atmospheric filtration at sunset or moon-set.

Pollution causes the visible light to turn orange or red due to the filtering effects of pollution on this light. The more pollution there is, the redder it will look. This can be seen on the Island of Hawaii where the Kilauea volcano is erupting and pumping out gasses into the environment. The sunsets on this island are red, like the color of blood.

This is a problem near the poles, due to the Sun being lower in the sky. The sunlight is subjected to much more filtration by the atmosphere for longer periods of time. This may be unhealthy for people who live nearer to the poles.

Filtering solar radiation with air pollution is a bad idea.

A good example of pollution in the atmosphere is on the cover of my first book "Solar Photovoltaic Design for Residential, Commercial and Utility Systems" which is shown in the next picture. This picture was taken from the summit of Kitt Peak National Observatory in Sells, Arizona. At an elevation of approximately 6,875 feet, we can see an orange sunset. This sunset several hundred years ago probably would have been a white sunset. Orange and red sunsets are characteristic of a polluted atmosphere. Viewing the midday Sun through smoke also produces an orange or red view of it.

Atmospheric Solar Filtering at Sunset

The orange sunset from Kitt Peak at 6,875 feet.

The next picture shows the effects of atmospheric pollution on the Sun. As you can see, it is a distorted view of the Sun. It is interesting that smoking causes cancer. Could it be that smokers are having cancer induced into them by the same effects as air pollution creates with solar radiation?

To ensure that you have good air quality in your home, you should check that you have a set of vents that allow air to come in from the outside of the home. One should be about one foot from the floor and the other should be about one foot from the ceiling on the opposite side of the home. This is to ensure that a cross flow of fresh, outdoor air is allowed to circulate within the home. The vents do not have to be large, but they should permit a fresh air exchange to occur continually within the home.

Outside your home, you should have a garden with lots of trees and plants. Trees and plants purify the air, helping to create the correct composition of air for the human.

"Our most basic common link is that we all inhabit this planet. We all breathe the same air. We all cherish our children's future. And we are all mortal."

John F. Kennedy

Atmospheric Pollution

Atmospheric pollution can cause Sun filtering and interference effects.

Water

You would think that water is one of the most understood subjects of human health, but it is not. This is evidenced by the many types of bottled water that are available at the supermarket. Water is marketed as mineral, reverse osmosis, steam distilled, distilled, vitamin, electrolyte, and so on.

In this chapter we will look into the inside and outside human water. Inside water is what you drink and outside water is what you bathe in. You will be surprised at how important water is for the human and also the ticking time bomb that you may create by not using the correct type of water.

Today, human survival on the Earth is almost completely dependent on the water tables around the world. Unfortunately, they are running out. Each year the water level is dropping and they are not being replenished. Instead, the trapped water is being released into the atmosphere where it is staying as water vapor.

This is a major problem for ground level solar radiation. Invisible water vapor appears to be raising the ground level solar radiation by lensing and interfering with the solar radiation from the Sun. This seems to have an effect in killing off some of the coral reefs in the oceans and possibly making some species of plants head towards extinction. The human race may already be heading down this route as well.

The only way that our planet can support the huge number of humans is due to the pumping of the underground water table. To stop using it means that we have to reduce the population size naturally at the earliest opportunity.

Trapped water is dead water. It may not have seen the surface of the Earth for a very long time. This is in contrast to river water that supports life within it. Trapped water has a very high mineral content associated with it. As

it starts to run out, it is highly likely that it will become toxic to humans.

Let us take a look at the different types of natural water:

- Rain is solar irradiated, radio frequency exposed, demineralized water with added nitrogen.
- River water is solar irradiated, grounded, mineralized water.
- Spring water is grounded, mineralized water.
- Sea water is solar irradiated, grounded, mineralized, high sodium water.

The human was drinking fresh river and spring water up until recently. Now let us see what the industrialized world calls water:

- Treated water.
- Particle filtered water.
- Carbon filtered water.
- Softened water.
- Reverse osmosis water.
- Steam distilled water.

Each of these is completely different from the other. It is somewhat ironic that the correct water to drink is the very first one, which is also known as "municipal water". It has plenty of minerals which the human body needs to extract from the water for the body to function correctly. It is unfortunate that fluoride may be added to the water supply which removes the choice of having it or not. Fluoride is a byproduct of the fertilizer industry and may

contain other toxic chemicals in it due to the way that it is produced.

The problem with filtered water is that you remove many of the particles that are present in it that the human body would either naturally use or reject. Filtered water may remove some of the organic nutrients that are actually useful to your body. You should remember that your body is equipped to drink natural untreated water, it has been doing it for thousands of years. You already possess an excellent water filtration system in your body, so this step at home is not needed.

Carbon filtering takes a lot of the chemical content out of the water. You may want to consider doing this if your water is known to be polluted but all municipal water has passed stringent tests to come into your home. You should only be carbon filtering water if you suspect that it needs to be done. Otherwise you are reducing the nutrient content of the water that you are feeding your body.

Softened water is a bad idea. Water softeners use a chemical ion exchange to change out calcium and magnesium ions for sodium ions. Sodium is salt, so you are changing your water from mineralized water to sodium water. You may get ill in the long term if you drank and bathed in this water. On the inside it is lacking essential minerals that your body needs and it has added sodium. On the outside it will start to strip minerals from your skin through osmosis. Chemically softened water does not occur in nature and you would be wise to avoid this type of water. If you were to water your plants with this water, then they may actually show stress and possibly die off. Some people who drink, bathe and shower in ion exchanged water react to it and will show skin rashes or itchy skin.

Water softeners are sold to people on the basis that it is better for washing clothes in and also protects your plumbing. The reality is that you may actually damage your plumbing, as softened water is unstable and wants to absorb minerals and it will do so by trying to extract them from your plumbing system. The same effect takes place in your body when you drink or bathe in it. You would not want to be exposing yourself to water that has extracted chemicals from your plumbing system.

Reverse osmosis water is promoted by many as being the same as rainwater. This is an incorrect statement as it is not the same as rainwater, it is just highly filtered and purified mineral water. It still does contain some contaminants, just in much lower numbers. Reverse osmosis is an extremely wasteful process with some units throwing way over 90% of the water to get less than 10% of usable water. It consumes a lot of energy as it needs pressure to push the water through the reverse osmosis filter membrane.

I have heard people call reverse osmosis water "*the best detergent know to man*" due to its ability to clean things. The reason why it is so good at cleaning is because it is unstable. The water is so clean that it wants to absorb the minerals around it to get back into the stable mineralized state. It will do the same with your body on both the inside and outside. You should avoid reverse osmosis water if you value your health.

Steam distilled water is probably the most expensive water that you can buy. It is what you are recommended to use in your steam iron to stop calcium deposits building up. This is the water that is most like rainwater. It is the purest man-made water generally available and I recommend that you only use it for the industrial purposes that it is recommended for. You should not be drinking or bathing in distilled water of any type long term.

Bottled water can be any of the above types. There is so much confusion regarding the labeling of bottled water that I recommend that you avoid it. Water cooler water that is in many offices has the same issues and I would recommend that you use municipal water for drinking due to the mineral content of it that your body requires. One of the major problems with bottled water is that it generally comes in plastic bottles. These bottles contain chemicals that can leach into the water over time and you may find yourself drinking some of the chemicals of the plastic as well as the water. These leached chemicals may impact your health later in life.

Softened, reverse osmosis and steam distilled water are all forms of de-mineralized water. It was shown back in the 1960's that the body actually appears to need hard water

so that it can extract the minerals from it. Lack of these minerals was found to cause heart arrhythmia. Many studies of hard water areas have found much lower incidences in cardiovascular diseases, cancer, respiratory diseases, diabetes and other health problems. When it comes to water, hard water is always your best choice for the human body.

Naturally occurring soft water does not have sodium ions as the chemical version does. It is soft because it is low on mineral content.

Drinking de-mineralized water regularly is known to cause acute health problems. This is due to calcium and magnesium being essential to the human body. The problems linked to low mineral intake are hypertension, coronary heart disease, gastric and duodenal ulcers, chronic gastritis, goitre, pregnancy complications and complications in infants.

We mentioned carbon filtering earlier. This is how trees and plants purify the water. A tree will absorb the water, store it, and slowly release it through its roots into the environment. Trees and plants are made of carbon, hence the carbon filtering that is prevalent in the water treatment industry. Water gets further filtration and mineralization through the soil before it gets into streams and rivers.

Swimming pools are an issue due to the chemicals that they contain. Every time that you swim in a swimming pool, you will be exposed to these. It is a well known problem in the industry and "Swimming Pool Cancer Risk" is extensively documented.

"Stray voltage" can be an issue around water and we will look into this later in the book.

Microwaved water is known for its toxicity. People have watered plants with microwaved water and have noticed that they tend to die! This is because the structure of the water has changed. Water structure is well known to be altered with light, sound, temperature, radio frequency, magnetic and electric fields. Some types of structuring are known for their health benefits, while others may make you sick. Human blood is 92%

water and you need to be careful how you let it be structured by external influences.

This is somewhat disturbing, given that the utilities are now installing high powered radio frequency transmitting devices onto domestic water supplies in the USA. Commonly called Smart/AMR/AMI utility meters, the utilities are now structuring the water that they are delivering to your home. The long term health effects of drinking such water is currently unknown at the time of writing.

Carbonated soft drinks should be avoided due to the carbonic acid that may damage the bones in the long term. Tea and coffee can act as diuretics and dehydrate you. The caffeine in them can upset your sleep cycles.

Testing of the various kinds of water led to the understanding that hot tea that had cooled had particularly beneficial effects on plants. It appeared to create resistance to radio frequency exposures. A daily pot of hot tea is likely to be beneficial to the human due to the nutrients that it contains. Outside of a daily pot of tea, you should be simply drinking municipal water. Drinking tea exclusively is known to create long term health problems. The radio frequency exposed, tea drinking Dieffenbachia plant is shown in the next picture alongside one that is only being given Tucson faucet water.

Tea Appears to Create Radiation Resistance

Watering a Dieffenbachia plant with hot tea that had cooled greatly improved its growth patterns in a radio frequency field when contrasted to the smaller and deformed Dieffenbachia plant that only got Tucson faucet water.

Gardeners have noticed that rainwater invigorates plants and it is likely due to this water being infused with nitrogen from the air and radio frequency exposed. Plants prefer to be watered through their leaves by this naturally treated rain water. Watering a plant with municipal water through its roots appears to be one of the reasons why you have to fertilize them.

A company called Vi Aqua (www.viaqua.com) markets a device that irradiates water with radio frequency at 27 megahertz. They claim that it extends the life of cut flowers and acts like fertilizer for plants, increasing the growth mass. They state the following effects have been observed in plants watered with radio frequency irradiated municipal water:

- **30% - 40% increase in crop size and yield.**
- **More disease-resistant.**
- **Require far less fertilizer.**
- **Need one third less water.**
- **Will thrive in poor soil.**
- **Taste better.**
- **Longer shelf life.**
- **Increases the solubility of nutrients in the water.**
- **Improves the quality of the plant and its lush appearance.**
- **Improves roots development.**
- **Optimizes the use of water by increasing its efficiency.**
- **Significant de-scaling effect in pipes and nozzles.**

What they have done is take an effect that is found in thunderstorms and apply it to groundwater. As can be seen, irradiating municipal water with radio frequency can accelerate growth and extend life. We also know that irradiating water with other frequencies can have detrimental effects.

A place where we find water in the human is in the amniotic fluid in the womb. Irradiating the womb with strange man-made frequencies would be expected to have an effect. Today, many women cannot give birth naturally to their babies because they are too big! Of those that do give birth naturally, they have a tendency to rip the vaginal canal due to the large size of the baby. It is quite possible that babies are significantly larger today because of man-made electromagnetic interference exposures! It may be the reason why they no longer fit into the birth canal in many cases. There is evidence in the historical records that indicates that birth weights increased after the introduction of the telegraph and electricity to the cities. The correct human birth weight appears to be in the 4 to 5 pound range. We know that delivering an oversized baby does damage to the birth canal and it is not recommended for good female health. Unfortunately, 6 to 10 pound babies appears to be a product of modern society.

Aaron Alexis, Navy Yard shooting suspect, thought people followed him with a microwave machine. He was actually correct in his assessment, as wondering around a modern city has you in high-powered microwave fields. You could be standing next to a high-powered cell phone microwave transmitter system and not even know it! Children in cities are noted for their accelerating development into puberty and irradiation of their body water by unnatural high-powered man-made radio waves is likely involved in this process.

You should avoid purchasing food and water from shops that are near to transmitter systems or that have wireless networking. It is likely that the food and water will have been structured and may have long term toxic effects to the human.

To sum up, the preference for good human health is to be drinking water that has been irradiated naturally by nature, not mankind.

"Water is the driving force of all nature."
Leonardo da Vinci

Food

Food is very well understood by humanity, but they just keep on ignoring the advice and eating foods from sources that should be avoided. Clearly a diet of fast food, genetically modified food, processed food, preserved food, and so on may make you ill eventually.

Organically grown fresh food is what you should be eating. The mix of food is generally incorrect and you should be eating a diet that consists mainly of fruits and vegetables. Meat and fish should probably comprise of less than 10% of your diet content. Fruits and vegetables are known for their antioxidant properties that prevent illness and disease.

Here is what you should be aiming for:

- **47% Vegetables.**
- **47% Fruits.**
- **3% Fish.**
- **3% Meat.**

You should realize that it is just a guide and feel free to indulge once a week in your favorite foods. A handful of nuts daily is a good habit, assuming you are not allergic to them.

The diagram on the next page shows the plant based food diet.

Plant Based Food Diet

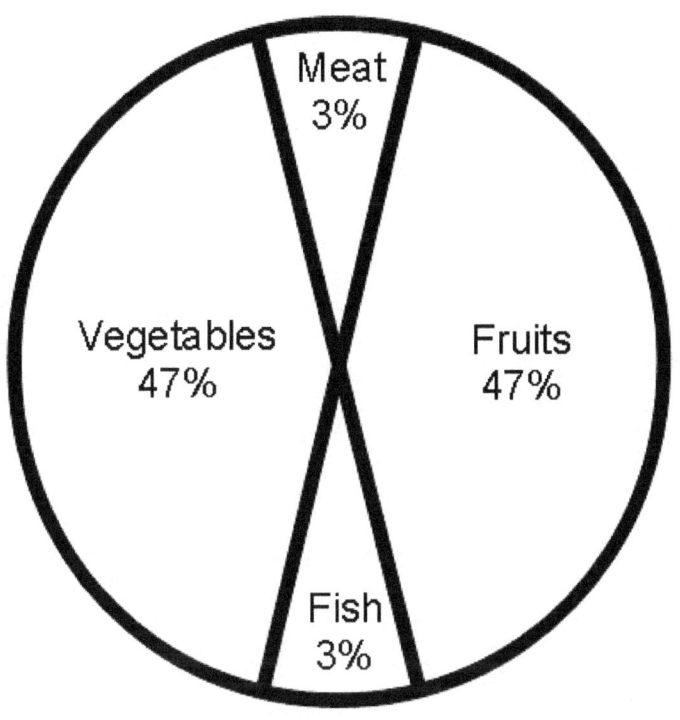

The adoption by many people of the "Atkins Diet" revealed problems in eating a diet that is largely comprised of meat. As the years passed, more health conditions were linked to this diet of high protein and fat intake. Some of these were:

- Coronary heart disease.
- Bad breath.
- Constipation.
- Dizziness.
- Headaches.
- Pregnancy issues.

Dairy is an unnatural food that humans should not be consuming. If you look at nature, there is no animal that consumes breast milk as an adult. The human is the only animal to do this, and it does it by drinking the breast milk of an entirely different species!

Calcium has long been quoted by the milk industry as an important aspect of health. Hard water and plant based foods contains all of the calcium that you will ever need as an adult! Instead of being led by biased advertising from the milk industry, you should follow what nature does:

Milk products should be avoided as an adult.

Modern humans have fat in common with diary animals. When you look at the fat cells of a modern human, they are the same color as the fat cells of diary cows. They are both yellow in color. This is in contrast to the fat on wild animals which is white. Both the modern human and the dairy cows lead similar lifestyles and it should be of no surprise to see that they share this feature. The reasons for this may be:

- Eating incorrect food.

- Exposure to the electrical system.

- Life under artificial lights.

- An indoor lifestyle.

- Disconnection from nature.

- Exposure to pollution.

- Lack of exercise.

- Loss of DC body voltage.

As people have started to realize, the modern human is a different creature from the human that lives a natural lifestyle in harmony with nature. People who are living in harmony with nature generally have little fat and it is white in color. You can tell the health of a person simply by the color of their fat. This fat effect was noted by Kevin Patterson in his book "Consumption".

Avoid being a fussy eater and eat everything on your plate. Use spices and sauces to give your food variety. Avoid having the same meal twice in one week. Pay attention to food that does not agree with your digestive system and may cause mouth or intestinal irritation to occur. Such foods should be avoided.

Being green on the inside is known to have protective properties to the human mind and body and you should aim for the majority of your diet to come from plant sources. NASA extensively uses fruit and vegetable based supplements to prevent cancer from occurring from Space radiation in the astronauts on the International Space Station.

"One cannot think well, love well, sleep well, if one has not dined well."

Virginia Woolf

Exercise

NASA has known for decades that if the astronauts do not exercise for approximately two hours per day when in Space that they will get sick. The top job an astronaut must do is exercise daily when on board the International Space Station!

Most modern humans now live in alien environments that are more comparable to Space than nature. Modern human environments are commonly devoid of trees and greenery. Instead concrete, paints and man-made materials predominate. The radiation levels have greatly increased with the advent of electricity and the associated products. Homes and workplaces are filled with electrical, electronic and wireless products. The environment in general is now heavily contaminated with wireless radiation that was not there even just a few years ago. The environment is overloaded with many wireless radiation sources.

To be healthy in modern society, you must adopt the behaviors of an astronaut!

NASA knows that sedate exercising, such as walking, does not work for the astronauts on the International Space Station. The exercise that they must do to stay in good health is vigorous exercise that strengthens the muscles throughout the body and makes them sweat! It is a tough job being an astronaut!

You are the equivalent of an astronaut living in modern society and you must copy what the astronauts are doing on the International Space Station in order to maintain good health. Daily high activity exercise is a must.

In order to do this I identified a workout DVD called "Supreme 90 Day System". The reason why I chose this DVD was because it was affordable, had great reviews, it converted fat to muscle mass and needed only a balance ball and dumb bells to perform the exercises at home. The exercises consists of ten routines of less than an hour each. They are relatively easy to do and get you sweating by the end of the routine.

I was quite shocked at how rapidly I saw the changes occurring. By the end of ten days, I had lost 6 pounds and my hunger had subsided. I was looking better and feeling great after the workouts. Clothes started to fit well and my health was improving. After twenty days my weight had stabilized, my muscle strength had greatly increased and the workouts were becoming routine and enjoyable. By thirty days my stamina had developed and I was able to fully perform each exercise routine.

It confirmed what I had been suspecting for quite some time, that walking is not really an effective exercise. I had been regularly walking for approximately an hour per day for exercise during the previous few years. When I started the workout DVD I was shocked at how unfit I had become!

When you are not exercising effectively every day, a process called "Muscle Atrophy" starts to take place. Every muscle that is not being used reduces in size. The process can be extreme in people who have had limbs immobilized through accidents or injury. Muscle atrophy is a wasting condition and it is highly undesirable to let your body go into this process.

Once the body has atrophied, you will become vulnerable to many conditions. This is because the human body was never meant to be in this condition. It is highly unnatural. The human spent thousands of years being active daily through hunting and gathering and your ancestors were really fit people! Modern society has brought with it sedentary lifestyles for the masses that are extremely unnatural. When man was a hunter gatherer, these atrophied humans would have been easy prey for any predator and atrophied humans were probably sparse. Muscle atrophy is not a natural state in the natural world and you should avoid entering into this condition.

I appeared to enter this condition when I started to work in desk jobs. This coincided with showing breathing difficulties and chest pains at the age of 37 when I was jogging in 2007. I did not know it at the time, but I had developed radiation sickness from working at high altitudes, sitting near to electrical rooms, exposure to electrical, electronic and wireless radiation emissions, and man-made ultraviolet light from florescent lights. Needless to say, once I started showing serious health conditions during exercise, I stopped jogging!

When I was researching why so many people were reporting reactions to radio waves, which is commonly called "Electromagnetic Hypersensitivity", muscle atrophy was one of my suspicions for it. Out of my family, I am the only one who does not exercise and I was the only person who was showing the sensitivity to wireless radiation. It appears that once the body has atrophied, then increased sensitivity to wireless radiation should be expected. This is because the electrical characteristics of the human body have changed. Muscle has very different electrical characteristics to fat.

You can buy devices that measure the fat content of the body using the principles of electrical conductivity. A fat human has a very different electrical conductivity to a muscular human. As such, the electrical properties of an atrophied human are very different to those of a muscular human. The electronic devices are commonly called "Body Fat Monitors" and use the principle of "Bioelectric Impedance Analysis (BIA)".

It appears that muscle atrophy puts the human into a zombie-like state that is unnatural. The body is not dead, but it is not fully alive either. This opens up the human for biological attack on many fronts. The natural world defines an atrophied human as weak and will target it. Your body was never meant to function in the natural world in an atrophied state.

Fortunately, muscle atrophy is easily avoidable and it simply requires that you do effective strength exercises daily. If you want to be healthy, you need to be in good physical condition with toned muscles. Human resources departments have known for a long time that people who look healthy and keep fit generally are the healthiest employees!

It is in your interest to be fit and strong. The health benefits far outweigh the time that it takes to keep yourself toned. Exercising will keep you in harmony with the natural world. Skin that is made to sweat eliminates toxins from the body in the process and cleanses the human. Exercise that makes you hot throughout is raising your core temperature and changes the cellular system environment in a positive way.

Muscle clearly has electromagnetic shielding properties for the human body. Physical exercise that causes the brain to move around will improve the supporting structure to the brain and may well increase its resistance to man-made electromagnetic radiation exposures. After six months of building muscle mass I can now confirm that muscle mass creates increased tolerance to biologically harmful radiation sources.

After six months of vigorous exercising to build muscle, my body is now lean. I combined this technique with creating a DC voltage on the human body and this has coincided with no longer observing the adverse reactions that I was displaying regarding continuous radio frequency exposures at my home. We will discuss the creation of the DC body voltage in the next chapter.

The elderly and infirm are typically in some state of atrophication. Unfortunately, babies and many modern children are in the atrophied state and this makes them vulnerable to radiation exposures. The environment that the next generation are being raised in is very unnatural and is hostile to atrophied youngsters. We will look into the rise of Autism in the children later in the book.

"Those who think they have no time for bodily exercise will sooner or later have to find time for illness."

Edward Stanley

Body Voltage

Most people associate direct current (DC) voltage with batteries. It has a constant voltage that does not change over time. What most people do not know is that the human is supposed to have a DC voltage on its body relative to its feet. This voltage is generated from both the atmosphere and nutritional intake.

Atmospheric energy has direct current in it and it has a voltage gradient that is positive relative to the ground in clear conditions. In cloudy conditions it is negative for the first couple of miles above the ground and that then changes to positive polarity as you go higher into the atmosphere. Close to the ground the voltage increase is between 1 to 19 volts per foot. Flying kites with conductive strings will expose you to this atmospheric voltage, as will helium balloons with long conductive strings. Higher up in the atmosphere, the voltage increases by approximately 30 volts per foot.

All living organisms that stand tall on the ground are subjected to this DC voltage and this is evidenced in the following pictures.

The Dieffenbachia grows well regardless of if the voltage is positive or negative 1.5 volts on its stem relative to the roots. It indicates that the atmospheric DC voltage polarity may reverse in nature over time. It seems that the atmospheric DC voltage in my area has changed, which is very concerning!

If the DC voltage gets too high, then the Dieffenbachia plant starts to show stress. 9 volts positive polarity on the stem appears to cause growth defects (shown) and seems more harmful than 9 volts negative stem polarity that seems to stunt growth and corrodes the metal alligator clip.

My plants are grown in high radiation fields that appear to come from radio frequency transmitting utility meters and three cell phone towers that are between 600-700 meters from my home. The Dieffenbachia's all deform at my home regardless of where they are grown at on my property. As we can see in the plants, we can restore the normal growth patterns by applying a DC voltage to them. The voltage has to be kept to the correct level, otherwise stresses will show up if too high or too low. Applying a DC voltage between the soles of the feet of the human and the upper body may have applications in the field of human health. This is shown in the next diagram.

I have been experimenting with putting the human mind and body into a DC electric field during sleep. I have a large sheet of conductive aluminum foil attached to the 10 feet high ceiling above the bed and a large sheet of conductive aluminum foil on the floor under the bed to effect this. The upper sheet is connected to the negative terminal of a battery and the lower sheet is connected to the positive terminal. This can be seen in the following photograph.

The upper sheet is akin to the tree canopy which is known to have a DC voltage on it. A company called Voltree Power (www.voltreepower.com) is developing the use of tree voltage to power electronic systems and has extensively researched the DC voltage of trees.

The feet are connected together through being in contact with the conductive ground and are earthed (grounded). The mind and body are walking around in a DC voltage field. That DC voltage will energize the mind and body and the lack of it may make the human sick.

Human Electrical Model

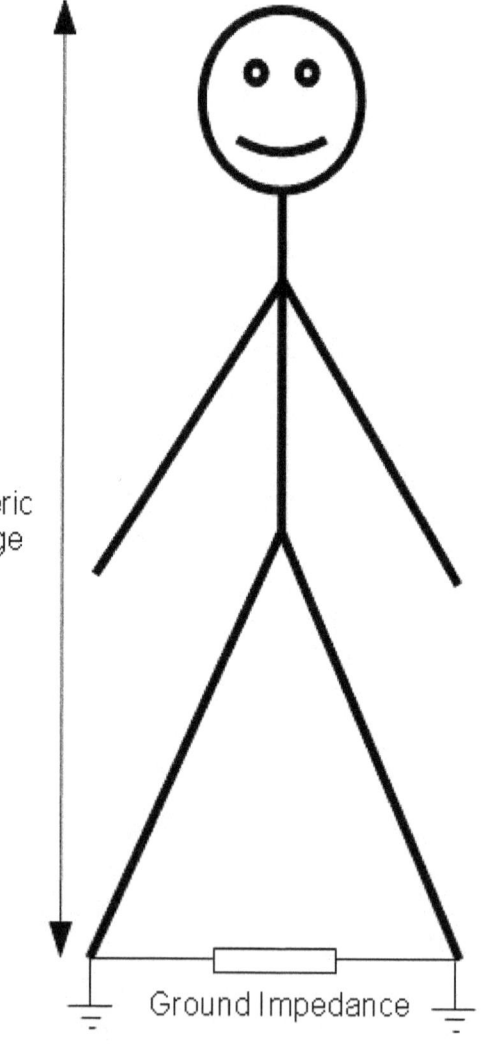

The upper and lower sheets of aluminum foil are the same size as the bed. The DC voltage on the conductive sheets will set up a DC voltage field between them with a small flow of energy that should pass through the human sleeping in the bed. This is currently an unproven experimental health technique that may have unknown side effects. I call this technique: "Electromagnetic Sandwich"

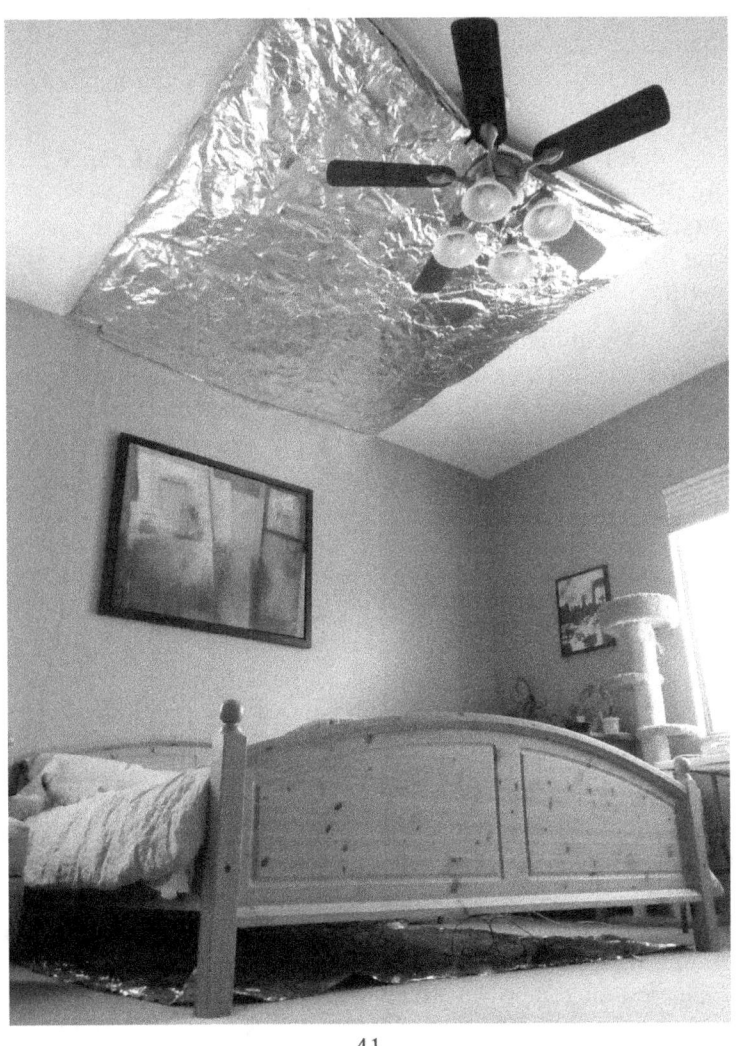

I started testing the Electromagnetic Sandwich with a 9 volt battery which should give approximately 2 volts of a negative atmospheric voltage exposure to my mind and body during sleep. The atmospheric voltage gradient between the floor sheet and the ceiling negative sheet is -0.9 volt DC per foot. I could definitely feel the difference when I was sleeping and headaches and muscle weakness showed up after about a week of testing. I changed the battery to 1.5 volt DC and found that this was much more agreeable to human health and the health problems cleared up. 1.5 volts DC appears to be more comparable to what you find on the tree canopy. I may adjust the DC voltage later, depending on what I find with long term testing.

It is interesting that the human health difference in the DC voltage exposures matches what I saw in the Dieffenbachia plants. Exposure to a very low DC voltage that is comparable to a single DC battery cell appears healthy for biological systems and 9 volts DC stresses them.

My initial assessment of the Electromagnetic Sandwich health technique was that the occasional daytime fatigue that I was experiencing significantly reduced. I find this very concerning, as it indicates that a DC atmospheric voltage is missing at my home that is required for both good plant health and good human health. It appears that people who suffer from Electromagnetic Hypersensitivity may be reacting to this loss of atmospheric DC voltage. They appear to be the electromagnetic radiation equivalent of the "Coalminers canary" and it is very foolish to ignore the health symptoms that these many people are reporting. They are very clearly reacting to unnatural man-made electromagnetic radiation conditions.

I further developed the Electromagnetic Sandwich technique for daytime use. It is easily implemented using an anti-static wrist strap and an anti-static mat. This is shown in the next picture. For those of you on the go, you can wear an anti-static heel strap and an anti-static wrist strap and just put the 1.5 volt DC battery in your pocket. Keep the cables as short as possible and it is preferable to use straight cables as opposed to the coiled cables shown in the picture. Long cables and cable coils act as antenna systems and will put strange frequencies onto the DC voltage that may lead to electromagnetic hypersensitivity.

These health techniques are experimental and have unknown side effects at the time of writing. The DC voltages may require adjusting to higher or lower levels and will be person dependent due to the impedance of the fat to muscle ratio. They may need to only be applied for short periods rather than continuous use. This is a developing area of research that is very new and there are a lot of unknowns currently.

If you choose to implement them, you should be under qualified and competent medical supervision and discontinue the techniques if adverse health symptoms show up. You would be assuming any and all risks using these health techniques.

When I discontinued the application of -1.5 volts DC from a single cell battery, I did develop a large withdrawal headache that slowly subsided over a few days. While I did initial testing with a negative body polarity, I currently recommend that a positive body polarity be used in the Electromagnetic Sandwich, as this appears to be what the body naturally produces, as we will see later.

Experimenting with wearing an anti-static strap on my wrist that is connected to the negative terminal of a 1.5 volt DC battery. The positive terminal is connected to an anti-static mat that my bare feet rest on. This creates a DC voltage gradient across my body that is similar to what nature does. Both the mat and the wrist strap have 1,000,000 ohm resistors built into them.

Zinc batteries are in common use, most disposable batteries that you buy for your products are zinc based. There are three types of zinc batteries and these are zinc-carbon, zinc-chloride and zinc-air. This is significant because the human body is made predominantly of carbon, through the lungs it absorbs air and chloride is salt that is present in the blood. So if you put zinc into the human body, you essentially create a zinc battery! It is widely recognized that the human mind and body functions on electricity and zinc is likely a key factor in this electrical functioning. It is clear from the plant experiments that wireless radiation is interfering with the DC voltage biological effects.

Natural sources of zinc are meat, poultry, diary products, beans, whole grains and nuts. You can create the zinc battery effect in the human body through zinc supplementation. You need to be careful with zinc supplementation as it may prevent copper absorption and you can overdose. Low level overdosing shows up as gastrointestinal symptoms and vomiting, severe overdosing can cause anemia, fever and central nervous system effects.

50% of zinc in the human body is found within the muscles. For this reason, you should ensure that you are muscular when in abnormal electromagnetic fields that are characteristic of modern cities. Muscles are the zinc batteries of the human body! Given that electromagnetic fields appear to deplete the zinc levels, you should be supplementing with zinc to replenish the levels when in a city environment.

All batteries are made from an electrolyte and at least two electrodes. The lemon battery is a good example of this. Inserting a piece of copper and a piece of zinc into a lemon creates the lemon battery. The lemon battery will generate a voltage of approximately 0.9 volts. This voltage can be increased by using magnesium in place of zinc. Magnesium and copper electrodes in lemons will generate approximately 1.6 volts DC. Many metals can be used to create the lemon battery, as can many fruits and vegetables.

The human is an electrolyte. The addition of metals to the human body will create the DC voltage effect. In 2013

Toxic Health © Steven Magee

I started to dose the human body with metal supplements to create metal electrodes within the body. The addition of salt increases the effectiveness of the body electrolyte. The voltage that I obtained after several weeks of dosing was in the range of +0.4 to +0.8 volts. These measurements were between the grounded feet and the tip of the finger or between the grounded feet the metal bridge in my mouth. The metal bridge always had the highest voltage and was approximately +0.2 volts higher than the finger tip. It was typical to see +0.5 volts on the finger tip and +0.7 volts on the metal dental bridge, relative to the grounded feet. These voltages were measured with an Amprobe 5XP-A multimeter.

The current produced was low and was about 5 microamps between the grounded feet and the finger tip. The current from the metal bridge to the grounded feet was much higher at up to 49 microamps. The voltage of the human body was always positive relative to the feet and this matches the atmospheric voltage in clear conditions. Given that the atmospheric voltage reverses in cloudy conditions, it may be related to the reason why so many people show depressive mood disorders in cloudy cities.

In nature, you would get the minerals and salts through your diet. In particular, coastal residents would be getting much higher levels of salts from their ocean based diet of fish and sea vegetables. The coastal Mediterranean lifestyle is associated with good health and is likely related to the optimum dosing of the body with metals and electrolytes through their diet.

It is likely that the body has the ability to be charged from the DC voltage in the atmosphere. In this situation, the grounded feet would form one plate of the battery and the skin of the body would form the other plate. Hair on the body likely increases the surface area of the skin to increase the effectiveness of the connection to the DC voltage in the atmosphere. This connection to the atmospheric DC voltage may facilitate the correct chemical composition of the electrolyte of the human body. Without the atmospheric DC

46

voltage, the human may slowly fall into sickness and perhaps onto disease and premature death.

The DC atmospheric voltage is heavily interfered with by radio frequencies, tall structures and towers, and it appears to be either significantly reduced or missing at my home. It has been noticed that corrosion is accelerated near to transmitter systems and it is likely related to this effect. Corrosion is strongly tied to DC galvanic effects. As we now know, reduction or loss of DC atmospheric voltage equates to accelerated corrosion, plant retardation and poor human health. It may also be related to climate change and extreme weather events.

As such, I have been experimenting with the following supplements to create the battery effect in the human body:

- Cobalt (B-12).
- Copper.
- Iron.
- Magnesium.
- Salt.
- Zinc.

The plagues of our children are Autism and Attention Deficit Disorder (ADD). Doctors have found that the following supplements reduce symptoms in these children:

Autism: Cobalt (B-12).
ADD: Magnesium and zinc.

The doctors who supplement children with these are unlikely to realize that they are creating a DC voltage on the human body. It is likely that the presence of the DC voltage is reducing these conditions.

When applying a DC voltage between the foot and the wrist, a reaction occurred in my urine. It started to smell like a strong chemical, similar to WD-40. I was concerned that this may have been a reaction to the battery and it was one of the reasons why I switched over to creating the DC voltage with supplements. After ceasing to apply the battery voltage, the chemical smelling urine disappeared after approximately one week. It reappeared shortly after supplementing for DC voltage. The chemical smelling urine lasted for a few months until finally reverting back to its normal smell. I am assuming that the DC voltage created a reaction in the body that was causing elimination of a stored substance that currently remains unidentified.

Another source of the above metal supplements is multivitamins. Multivitamins are a minefield and you should not go out and buy them unless you know what supplements that you require. Many people have made themselves sick by using the wrong multivitamin formulation. The next time you are in the supermarket, pick some different brands of multivitamins up and read the supplement information. They will likely all be very different from each other.

If you are suffering from radio frequency exposures, then the electrolytes and metals appear to offer good resistance to them. Given the large scale deployment of radio frequency producing devices over the last decade, it is likely that you may have conditions that are related to these exposures. Accelerated metal corrosion has been widely observed near to radio frequency transmitters and it is probable that it also corrodes the metals within the human body. Reduction of the body metals may result in a reduction of the DC body voltage which may lead to sickness.

When supplementing, I would recommend that you check out the reviews for the supplements that you are planning on taking to ensure that people are having success with them. Everyone is different and what works for one may not work for another. Different brands may use different sources for their supplements and comparable supplements may have contrasting effects due to manufacturing differences. You should consult with your doctor regarding the correct supplements to take.

I currently supplement daily with the following to create the DC voltage on the human body:

B-12: 500 mcg

Copper: 2 mg

Iron: 25 mg

Magnesium: 250 mg

Zinc: 19 mg

Salt: 1,000 mg

Comparable formulations may be found in some multivitamins. I have found that my overall health has increased since supplementing and this is in line with the DC voltage and currents that have appeared during that time. Supplementing with other additional metals may increase the beneficial effects of the DC voltage. You will need to discuss an appropriate supplementation dose with your doctor if you choose to do this.

A word of warning: I originally took the metal supplements separately every two hours during the daytime. So the first metal was taken at 08:00, the second at 10:00, the third at 12:00, and so on until I had taken all of the different supplements for the day. This had the very interesting effect of making my brain functioning go very weird, confused and forgetful! It appeared that I had created a DC battery within the intestines!!! Striping of the intestines with different metals is very undesirable and matches the findings that human brain functioning and intestinal health are strongly linked. Taking all of the supplements together at breakfast remedied the brain problems.

I saw my mating cycle get triggered when taking high doses of zinc during developing the metal supplementation techniques. It was likely a reaction to the rapidly changing DC voltage levels. Too much daily zinc eventually led to a metallic taste in the mouth, runny nose, sore throat and fatigue. This led to me reducing the dosage.

I saw headaches develop initially when supplementing with salt. This was accompanied by nerve twitching. It cleared up after approximately a week.

My thyroid became sore and it was difficult to swallow during the initial few months of DC supplementation. It felt like a lump in my throat, although to the touch there was nothing there. It subsided to the just the right side of my thyroid and then eventually disappeared.

Introducing metal supplements into the human body is likely to increase the electromagnetic shielding effects. It appears that a human who is supplementing with metals becomes more resistant to radio frequency exposures.

I have tested two multivitamins that are branded "Energy". I never noticed much difference with either when compared to the supplements that I use for DC voltage. Going into rural areas, beaches and the countryside is the most effective energy supplement that I have found and this is line with the cities being filled with excessive radio frequency energy which is well known to induce fatigue into many people.

I call supplementing with electrolytes and metals:

The Electrical Chemistry of the Human

It is my conclusion that the human mind and body is essentially a single cell rechargeable battery that is charged from the atmospheric DC voltage and the Earth. When in areas where the atmospheric DC voltage is reduced or missing, the human slowly discharges and becomes sick. The human can be recharged either by going into rural areas where the atmospheric DC voltage is still intact, or by connecting a single cell battery between the soles of the feet and the wrist, or by ingesting electrolytes and a wide range of

metal supplements. Human battery discharge rates appear to increase if the person has metal implants. Human mind and body metals appear to be lost through radio frequency exposure and I call this hypothesis:

Internal Human Corrosion

Internal human corrosion that leads to the loss of human DC voltage appears to be a slow form of electrocution that may lead to premature death over many decades. It may be also caused by metal implants in the body. Self discharge of batteries typically occurs at rates of 8% to 20% per year and the human may display similar discharge rates. Discharge occurs due to internal currents within the battery. If the human is not charged daily from the atmospheric DC voltage and the ground, then complete DC discharge may eventually occur and the human essentially becomes a flat battery.

For more information on body voltage, I can recommend the following books

"Healing is Voltage" by Jerry Tennant.

"The Body Electric: Electromagnetism And The Foundation Of Life" by Robert Becker.

"We cannot hope to either understand or to manage the carbon in the atmosphere unless we understand and manage the trees and the soil too."

Freeman Dyson

Smells

One of the things that you will notice when in a forested environment are the smells! Everything around you will be releasing scents and pollen into the air. Plant scents and pollen may be essential to good human health! The nose and lungs extract the scents and pollen for use in the human body.

The other thing you will notice when you look at modern society is the large number of people who have allergies. This is not normal. Clearly, we are a species that lived in the forest until a few hundred years ago and we were not allergic to it. Allergies are a result of a modern industrial society. It is far more likely to be related to the stress placed onto the body by living in an unnatural environment.

With each change that the modern human has made to its environment, new stresses were introduced. This build up of stresses leads to a poorly functioning human. Once the human is in the poorly functioning state, it becomes prone to illness and disease. Allergies are one of the signs of this poorly functioning state.

Exposure to pollen may be needed to be in a healthy state and you should be querying why you are allergic to something that humans have lived in the presence of for thousands of years. It is most likely that something in your environment is making your body react to it. If you have gone into pollen deficiency, then the adverse reaction to the arrival of higher pollen levels is normal and the best way to deal with it is to actually increase your outdoor time in natural green environments! Your body should adjust to the presence of pollen within a few weeks.

Avoiding pollen when your body is pollen deficient is a bad idea and will only make matters worse. Unfortunately, it is very easy to become pollen deficient in a city environment with the lack of nature in the area. The sealed up, air conditioned homes just add to the problem of pollen

deficiency. **Smart people keep their windows open, have plants inside, gardens outside, and spend daily outdoor time in the nearest natural green environment with trees.**

Outdoor smells change with the seasons and also with humidity. You will notice that during and after rains that you will be smelling air that is infused with nature!

Modern homes are connected into sewer systems. You need to be careful with your sewer system as it has the potential to fill your home with sewer gas! Sewer gas is poisonous and explosive. If homes in your area start to mysteriously explode, it is likely that the sewer system is aging and has started to leak sewer gas into the home.

Sewer gas is generally noticeable when coming into the home from outdoors after the home has been locked up for several hours. If you enter the home and notice a strange smell, then it is likely that your sewer line is leaking somewhere inside the home. Things that can cause this are:

- Drains traps have dried out.
- Toilet drain wax seal is leaking.
- Cracked drain.
- Kitchen island vent valve is leaking.
- Dishwasher or washer needs to be run.

All drains should have water flushed through them at least twice a week to prevent them from drying out and leaking sewer gas into the home. They rely on the presence of water to seal the drain. Your washer and dishwasher should be run at least twice per week to prevent any water inside of it going moldy and emitting spores.

The guest bathroom is particularly hazardous for single people and couples. If you have guests infrequently, then the drains in that room are likely to dry out and vent the sewer system gas into your home! You should make a point of regularly going into this room and flushing all of the drains with water to ensure that they are sealed.

You should pay attention to how your home smells when entering it. It is good practice to take a big sniff of the air every time you enter the home. Strange smells should be tracked down. Low levels of sewer gas smell like rotten eggs and high levels can destroy your sense of smell. The symptoms to look for are:

- Extreme fatigue.
- Dizziness.
- Headaches.
- Irritability.
- Memory loss.
- Runny eyes.
- Runny nose.
- Excitation.
- Rapid breathing.
- Headaches.
- Seizures.
- Loss of consciousness.
- Coma.
- Death.

Out-gassing can be a problem and is noticeable around new products. Most people associate it with the new car smell. That new car smell is the products releasing gasses into the car from the chemicals that were used to make it. You generally notice out-gassing in the home whenever you bring a new item into the home, such as a new sofa or mattress. It is important to ventilate your home well

during the few weeks after introducing a new item into the home. If your home is exhibiting the new car smell, then you should have your windows open.

Out-gassing is noticeable for a few weeks after introducing a new product. Over time the product will release less gas and the new smell will slowly subside. Many products will continue to out-gas indefinitely, but the volume of gas is low that they emit. It is for this reason that you should ensure that your home has adequate outdoor ventilation installed into it to enable the out-gassing to escape into the outdoors. This is a concern due to the human body constantly extracting nutrients from the air.

Basements are an issue due to most toxins being heavier than air and they will accumulate in the lowest area of the home. You should avoid spending extended time in basements as they generally have the most toxic air in the home. If you do spend extended time in a basement, then you should ensure that there is a source of fresh air coming into the area.

For those of you with indoor cats, you should be changing out the cat litter regularly. Keep the cat litter at the furthest point from the bedrooms and get into the habit of checking it several times per day.

Make sure that your kitchen trash can seals in the smells and empty it daily. Keep it near to an outdoor air vent.

It is important to pay attention to the smells in your home and I do recommend the installation of an upper and lower air vent in every home to facilitate an exchange of outdoor air into the home. If you are breathing stale air due to lack of ventilation, then you may start to get sick.

"The flower that smells the sweetest is shy and lowly."
William Wordsworth

Temperature

The optimal temperature for the human body appears to be around 70 to 80 degrees Fahrenheit. It is interesting to note that the temperature of the forest floor in the tropics is a stable 72 degrees Fahrenheit. Research for this book is indicating that this is the correct human environment for excellent health.

If you go below 70 degrees Fahrenheit, you will get cold and start to shiver if you do not put clothing on. Above 80 degrees Fahrenheit you will start to get hot and fatigued.

Humans have developed heating and cooling systems to enable them to live anywhere that they want to. Exposure to these systems is likely to have health implications by cycling your temperature up and down, between indoor and outdoor environments. It is better to live in a location that is in harmony with your body and does not require artificial systems to keep you comfortable.

Two story homes should be avoided with heating and cooling systems. They typically end up with a hot upstairs and a cool downstairs. It is impossible to get an even temperature throughout the home. Single story homes do not exhibit this problem.

When you look into the native people in the Southwest USA, you notice that they were nomadic. They would live in the mountains where it was cooler in summertime and relocate to the lower elevations in wintertime where it was warmer. Nature provides the correct human environments all year round, you just have to follow them!

Plants are the same. Seeds only germinate in a narrow range of temperatures. If the temperature changes and is outside of this range then germination will not occur. As you can see, temperature is very important in plants too!

As the temperatures change around the globe in response to climate change, we will see a great change in the range and species of all life around the world. There is a possibility that it will eradicate humanity if the shift in temperature is too large in either direction.

People have long associated health conditions with changes in temperature. Arthritis is well known for people to report pains when the weather goes cold. Many arthritis sufferers develop an uncanny ability to predict the weather!

"Even if temperatures and conditions went flat from this point forward, we anticipate that Arctic ice would eventually disappear."

Ted Scambos

Humidity

Humidity is very important in human health and it is the amount of water vapor in the air. Too much or too little can be undesirable. The ideal level of humidity appears to be about 35% to 50% for excellent human health.

Low humidity typically occurs in winter when you heat your home. The heat reduces the humidity levels. Low humidity can bring:

- Sore throats.
- Sinus pains.
- Dry skin.
- Chapped lips.
- Itchy eyes.
- Excessive thirst.
- Static discharges.

You can bring up the humidity levels in your home by using a humidifier. Too much humidity can bring:

- Sweating problems.
- Breathing problems.
- Condensation.
- Dust mites.
- Mold.
- Mildew.
- Fungus.

- Spores.
- Musty smells.
- Wood will expand and windows and doors may stick.

Everything will have a damp feel to it. It is a good reason not to buy homes that are frequently in clouds or fog. If humidity levels get too high in the home, then you can bring them down by using a dehumidifier.

"Know how weather, especially humidity, can affect the movement of doors and windows."

Marilyn vos Savant

Light

You would think that after thousands of years of studying the Sun, we would know everything there is to know about light but this is not the case. Light is only just starting to be understood in the human environment.

The many types of light appear to be able to induce the symptoms of Electromagnetic Hypersensitivity (EHS) into the human mind and body. Light is part of the electromagnetic spectrum and it should come as no surprise that it is able to induce similar problems that other types of radiation can produce in the human body.

One of the things that had me a little confused when researching this section of the book was the symptoms of Electromagnetic Hypersensitivity (EHS) occurring without the presence of electrical and electronic equipment. I later realized that there is no place on Earth that is free of man-made electromagnetic radiation with the advent of ground based radio and microwave transmissions and later, Space satellites that are routinely beaming electromagnetic energy to the surface of the Earth.

The types of man-made electromagnetic radiation are shown on the next page.

This makes it somewhat difficult to research the natural human solar radiation environment, as it is no longer natural! When outside, you are now subjected to a wide range of man-made electromagnetic frequencies that were not there just a few years ago. The man-made electromagnetic spectrum is increasing on a daily basis as the human addiction to modern technologies continues to gain momentum.

At the same time as the use of technology is increasing, we are witnessing the rise of human illness, cancer and the shortening of the human lifespan. They are all connected and it would be foolish to ignore this fact. Indeed, in 2011 the link between cancer and cellphones has become established. Cellphones in the future may be viewed the same way that asbestos and cigarettes are today.

Aside from the soup of man-made electromagnetic radiation that we now find ourselves immersed into, we have changed the atmospheric gas composition drastically over the last few hundred years of the Industrial Revolution. This is commonly referred to by many as the carbon levels rising in the atmosphere. They are approximately at double the levels recorded in the historical records and there are no doubts that the use of fossil fuels to drive the Industrial Revolution caused this to occur.

So why is this a problem for solar radiation? Well, it is not just the levels of carbon that went up, it is the levels of almost everything else that went up too! There is far more water vapor stored in the atmosphere from the over use of modern crop farming techniques that use irrigation, and this is just one of the many examples of things that have changed the atmospheric gasses. The problem with far more molecules in the atmosphere is that they will do a number of things:

- Block the Sun's rays.
- Heat up.
- Start moving more energetically.

- Create solar radiation interference effects.

- Interference effects may lead to illness, disease, cancer and premature death in humans, and throughout the natural world.

But it does not stop there. The addition of certain chemicals to the atmosphere will destroy wavelengths of light and it may only be a matter of time before one of these wavelengths of light that is critical for human survival is eliminated. This is called:

The Extinction Wavelength

The extinction wavelength of light may be achieved in the near future that could lead to the mass extinction of the human race. So, for sunlight and human health, atmospheric pollution is an extremely serious problem! It is entirely possible that we may achieve the extinction wavelength within the next fifty years and that will mark the start of the end for humanity.

Looking at the diagram on the next page, we can see that the atmosphere is already removing parts of the solar radiation spectrum at sea level. This wavelength reduction effect is at its worst in polluted cities, especially ones nearer to the poles.

With each passing year the solar radiation spectrum is slowly changing. As the atmosphere fills up with molecules from pollution we will move towards increasing filtering and interference effects from the Sun. Increased sunlight filtering and interference is likely to increase the disease rates in all living organisms, including the human.

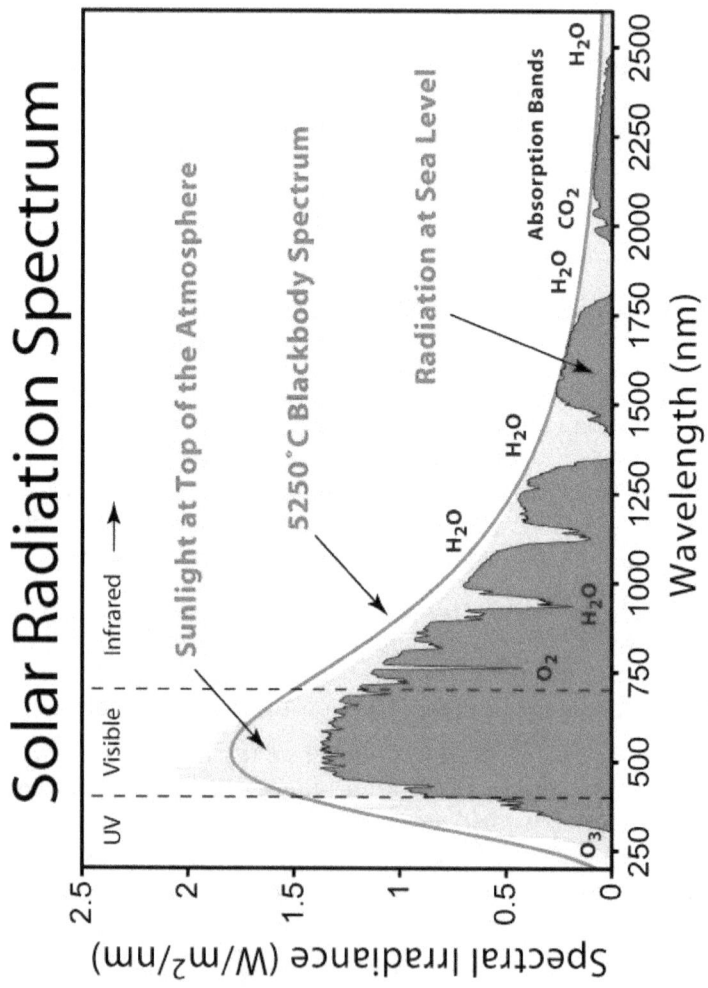

We can see this effect in plants. Plant leaves change with different solar radiation levels. The same plant will change the color, shape and size of the leaves to match the level of solar radiation that it receives. There is a limit to how adaptable each plant is and if the radiation gets outside of its range, the plant will start to show stress and may die.

Photosynthesis also occurs in the human body when it is exposed to sunlight. The latest research is indicating that the photosynthesis effects that take place within the human mind and body are extensive and wide ranging, and that vitamin D production is just one small part of it. Light has major functions in:

- **Modulating heart rate.**
- **Circadian rhythms.**
- **Digestion.**
- **Hormones.**
- **Mood.**
- **Fear.**
- **Mental state.**
- **Blood.**
- **Skin.**
- **Bone development.**
- **Mental development.**

Some of the ports of entry of natural light into the human body are:

- **Skin.**
- **Ears.**
- **Eyes.**

- **Nose.**
- **Lips.**
- **Nails.**

Painting nails is a human habit that may cause damage to the human body by covering up the blood that is circulating in the nail bed. Using lipstick may have the same effect on the blood circulating in the lips. It will prevent this blood from being irradiated by the Sun.

Is the wet surface of the eye providing regulation to the blood plasma? Irradiation of the saline solution of the eye may be essential to the proper functioning of the blood plasma.

Hair creates interference effects that modify the sunlight to an interference form of light. Dr. John Nash Ott noted that when he started to spend the majority of his time outdoors that his thinning hair started to regrow! Indeed, the hair regrowth industry markets ultraviolet and infrared light treatments as hair regrowth products. You do not need to purchase these products, as nature provides the treatments for free! Simply by spending time outdoors in the shade of trees should stimulate the hair regrowth effect.

The human mind and body may need to receive sunlight through the tree canopy in order to be in a healthy state. I call this light "Interference Green Light" and it may be the top thing that you need to be receiving in order to be in good health and free of pain. It is very different from direct sunlight due to:

- A much lower power level.
- It is filtered.
- It has interference.

Unfortunately in modern society, there are a large number of people who are sunlight deficient. This occurs through the use of cars, homes, offices, indoor shopping, and so on. The importance of getting daily Sun exposure has been lost on the modern generation and it is making them ill in large numbers.

Daily irradiation of the human mind and body by natural sunlight is an extremely important aspect of human health.

So how much sunlight should you aim for every day in order to be healthy? It is unique to each person. Typically a person with light skin needs less time and a person with dark skin needs more time outdoors. You should aim to spend as much of your day as possible outside in a natural environment, preferably in the shade of the tree canopy.

Toxic light presents a hazard to human health. There are many sources of toxic light and you should learn to recognize these sources. Potentially toxic light is almost everywhere in modern society:

- Artificial street lighting.
- Artificial home lighting.
- Artificial office lighting.
- Anywhere where there is glass.
- In your car.
- In your home.
- In your office.
- Televisions of every type.
- Computer monitors of every type.
- At sunrise.
- At sunset.
- Near the north and south poles.
- In any large city.

- In chemical trails from aircraft.

- In polluted atmosphere.

- Anywhere where the tree canopy is not present.

So what may toxic light be shown to do in the future? In the future the following conditions may be proven to be related to toxic light:

- Developmental problems.

- Cancer.

- Depression.

- Heart attacks.

- Circulation issues.

- Diabetes.

- Brain and nerve issues.

- Disruption of circadian rhythm.

- General aches and pains.

- Aggression.

- Psychiatric problems.

- Many of the current medical problems in society may be related to toxic light.

Humans tend to develop their land with modern agriculture and construction techniques which are not conducive to the natural world. It is ironic that through this unnatural development of their land that modern humans actually create environments that are unhealthy for them. Humans who develop their land in unnatural ways, such as clearing, introducing modern farming techniques, paving with concrete, and building tall structures really should not be surprised if their health deteriorates and they die prematurely.

Light sources come in many forms and here is a list in the order of quality of light:

- Under the tree canopy:
    - The best form of light for the human mind and body.
- Direct sunlight:
    - You need to be careful of this form of light as it is very powerful and may burn you. You can damage your eyes in this environment.
- Behind glass:
    - Glass filters light and removes wavelengths of light. Many types of glass excessively filter light to create a toxic form of light to the human mind and body.
- City sunlight:
    - The cities have many tall buildings that raise the radiation levels around them. The solar radiation levels in cities can be very high, have modified spectrums, and are extremely unpredictable.
- Artificial light:
    - Artificial lighting is not full spectrum daylight and may cause illness in the human mind and body.
- Office lighting:
    - This tends to be florescent lighting and is produced by just a few colors of wavelengths of light. It has a very spiked spectrum which does not occur in nature. The electronics that control them may emit electromagnetic interference (EMI).
- TV and computer monitors:
    - These tend to produce their colors from red, green and blue light and it is a very unusual spectrum

which does not occur in nature. The light is similar to florescent lights. The electronics that control them may emit electromagnetic interference (EMI).

- Street lights:
  - Street lights are predominantly gas discharge lighting and this is one of the most toxic forms of lighting to the human mind and body. The light tends to be monochromatic and they have problems with emitting electromagnetic interference (EMI).

- Neon signs:
  - These tend to have similar problems as streetlights.

You should be careful when choosing a home to live in and pay close attention to the location of streetlights. Streetlights can emit large amounts of electromagnetic interference, especially so when they switch on and also when they start to fail. The light also tends to be monochromatic and this type of light was shown by Dr. John Nash Ott to be harmful to biological systems. Indeed, I have noticed a trend in people who have died prematurely young and the presence of streetlights outside of their properties. The toxicity of streetlights has increased now that wireless transmitters are being installed into them.

The next diagram demonstrates the toxic effects of street lights. Electromagnetic interference (EMI), earth stray voltage, and stray currents will be looked into later in the book.

The following picture shows city nighttime light pollution in action. This area in San Diego is like daytime!

Streetlight Electromagnetic Interference

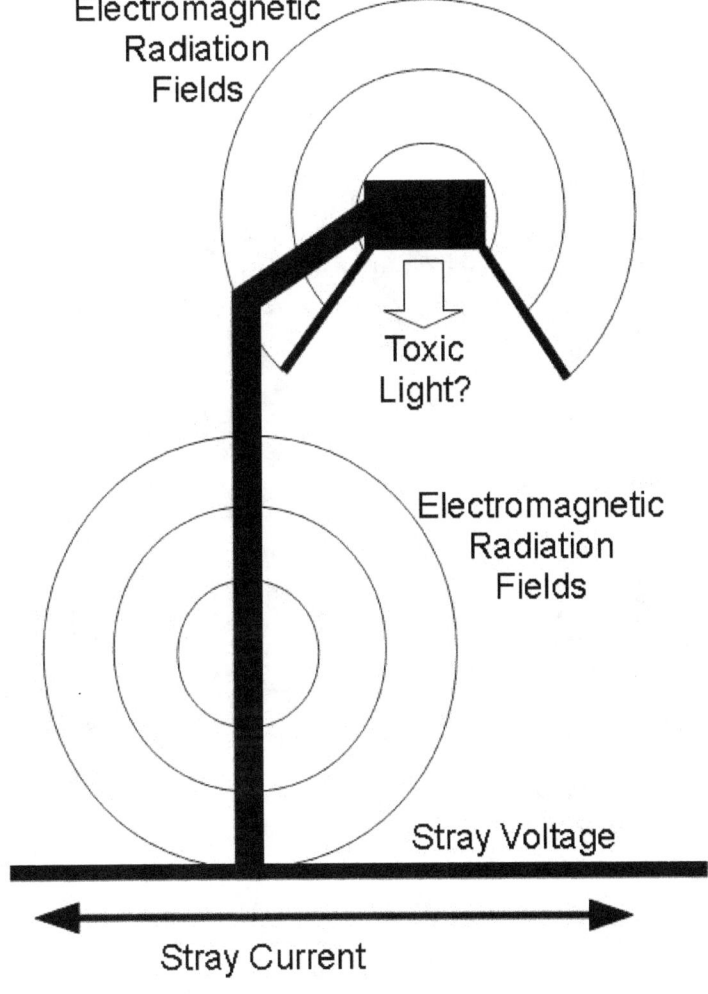

Electromagnetic
Radiation
Fields

Toxic
Light?

Electromagnetic
Radiation
Fields

Stray Voltage

Stray Current

City Streetlights

This is a picture of nighttime in San Diego, California. The light pollution is evident and may be harmful to human health in the long term.

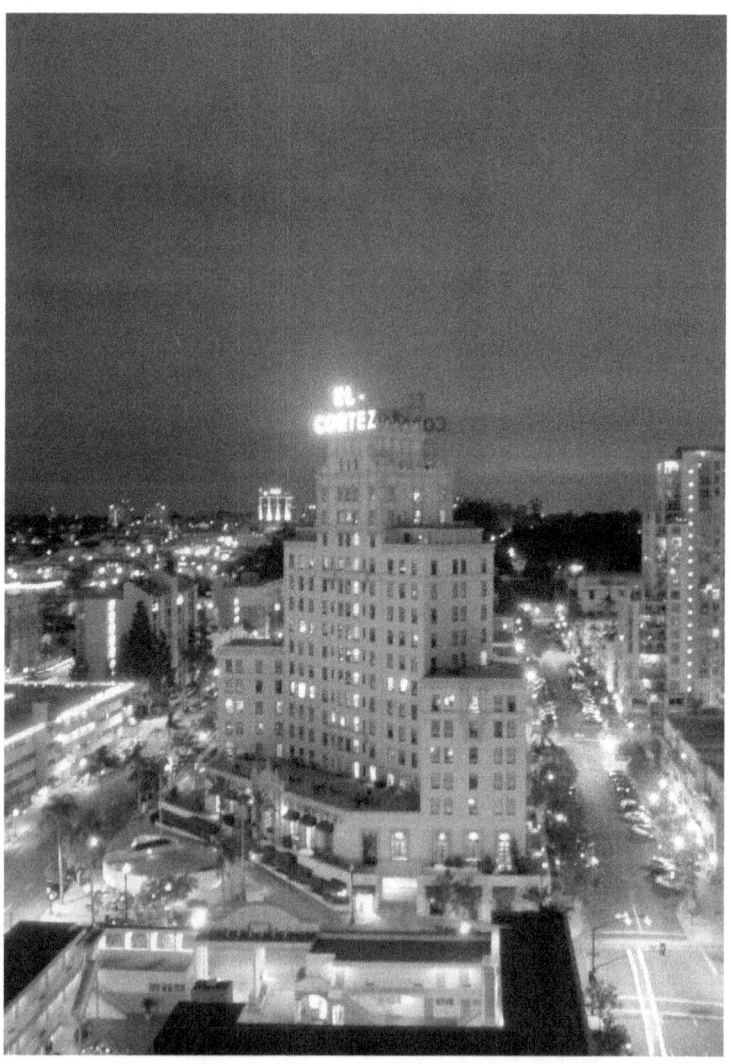

If you look at the next picture, it shows an effect that the tree canopy makes when solar radiation passes through it. This effect is called "Tree Canopy Light Interference". Light interference is a very big area of research in the optical and astronomical communities currently, it just has never been applied to the tree canopy.

Light is made up from waves and these waves can interfere with each other when passed through multiple apertures. The tree canopy makes many apertures that create the light interference effect. The result of this is that the solar radiation under the tree canopy is very different from the solar radiation above it. It is as different as night is to day.

The same effect occurs in water. The ripples on the surface of the water distort the light and create reflected interference light above the water and lensed interference light below the surface.

The interference wave diagram on the following page shows how the effect occurs.

Airy Disk Diffraction by Trees

The trees appear to produce the "Circle of Life" through tree canopy light interference.

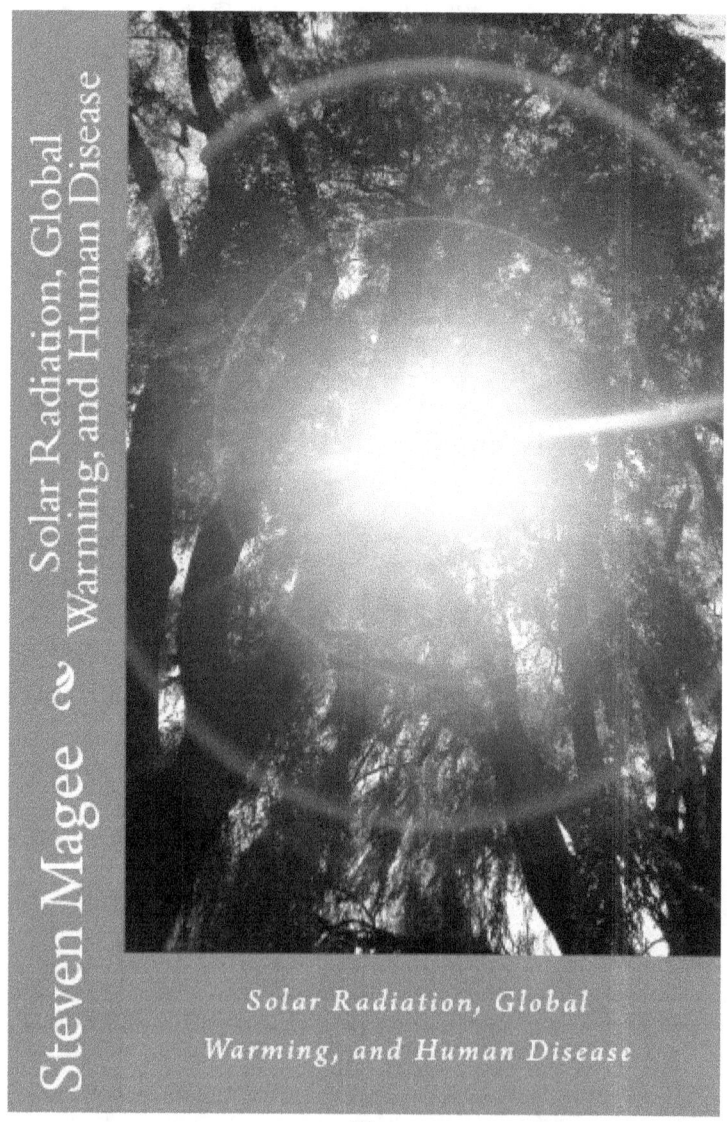

Light Interference Diagram

The light waves arrive in parallel and expand outwards when they pass through the two apertures. Interference is produced where the waves intersect. This is seen as the bright and dark bands on the right. The dark is destructive and the bright is constructive interference.

For more information on interference:
http://electron9.phys.utk.edu/optics421/modules/m5/Interference.htm

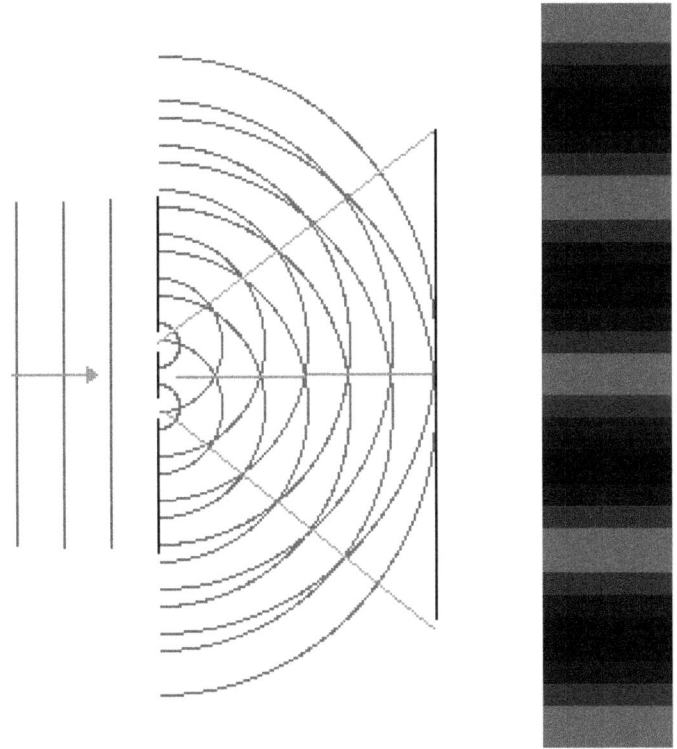

Interference of solar radiation may be caused by sunspots. Dr. Maki Takota showed that the presence of sunspots was related to the formation of certain chemicals in the blood. He also was able to relate blood chemistry to eclipses, solar flares, and sunrises.

A.L. Tchijevsky, a Russian professor, found a correlation between sunspot activity and human behavior. He linked major world events to the cycles of the sunspots! Generally, unrest was linked to sunspot maximum.

Sunspot minimum was linked to the occurrence of diseases in society by Professor d'Arsonval and others. It is not just human disease, crop production is affected too! Crops have a lower yield generally in sunspot minimum periods.

We really should not be surprised that sunspots can create changes in the human mind and body, as we have lived in the presence of the Sun for many thousands of years.

Sunspots do not cause much of a variance in solar irradiance levels from the Sun, typically oscillating up and down by just 1 watt per meter squared. It does not sound like much, but over the surface of the Earth, it is a huge amount of energy! The sunspot cycle is approximately eleven years and has been extensively studied by astronomers.

The picture on the next page shows the sunspot cycle and how the power levels vary.

Unfortunately, it appears that little attention was paid to the sunspot effect during the development of the Space industry. We now have an Earth that has thousands of man-made satellites circling it. Every time one of these passes in front of the Sun, it creates a man-made Sun spot! The effects of this are currently unknown on the human mind and body.

Aircraft create a similar effect when they pass in front of the Sun. Unfortunately, they also leave a chemical trail behind them that may linger for hours. The chemical trail will act as a filter to the sunlight and may also create interference effects.

The diagram on the next page shows satellite or airplane interference effects on the Sun. The following photograph shows the effects of aircraft chemical trails on the Sun.

Satellite Interference

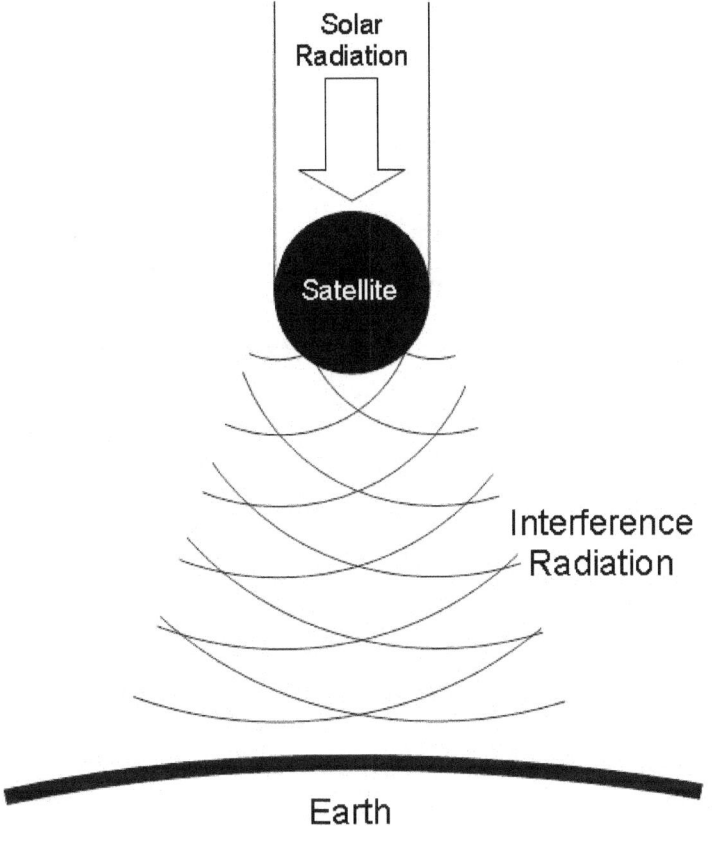

Aircraft Chemical Trails

The Sun as viewed entering an aircraft chemical trail. Many
groups have shown up around the world, protesting the
contamination of the sky and the strange optical effects that are
clearly visible. Many people who live in such areas now relate
their health problems to these effects.

Dr. Abraham Hoffer was able to link the human mental state to sunlight and, in particular, the equinoxes and solstices. He found that mental functioning peaks in January and July, and normalizes after March and September.

Trees absorb the majority of the solar radiation and only reflect a small percentage of it back into the environment. They also change the color temperature and spectrum of the solar radiation. To sum up, here are the effects that the tree canopy has on solar radiation:

- **Interference of solar radiation.**
- **Significant reduction in the power level of solar radiation.**
- **Create a stable power level of solar radiation.**
- **Color temperature modification of solar radiation.**
- **Spectrum modification of solar radiation.**
- **Conversion of solar radiation into natural energy.**

Without the tree canopy reducing and modifying the solar radiation, humans are subjected to flicker. This is an effect that is happening at sub-second speeds that is not noticed by the human eye. However, a high speed camera that shoots several frames per second can see this occurring. The Sun is basically increasing and decreasing its intensity due to atmospheric distortions and interference. Astronomers know this effect as "Astronomical Seeing". This effect may be able to induce dizziness, fatigue, headaches, epilepsy and nausea. Modern flicker may be a consequence of atmospheric pollution and may be far more severe than in the past.

An effect that is similar to this is broken clouds passing in front of the Sun. These produce extreme power cycles in the solar radiation levels. The power levels can change by over 90% very quickly. The human mind and body appears to have problems with this high level of

frequent power cycling and again may experience dizziness, fatigue, headaches, epilepsy and nausea.

Solar radiation is made up of direct, diffuse and albedo radiation power levels. Direct is the view of the Sun's disk, diffuse is the sky in general (the blue and cloudy part) and albedo is the reflections. Of these, direct contains over 90% of the energy, diffuse contains under 10%, and there is no limit on the power level that the albedo can be at. In a modern environment, such as a city, the reflections can increase the power levels many times higher than the sky based solar radiation of direct and diffuse combined.

Dr. John Nash Ott found that increasing the ultraviolet energy content of light can cause cells to rupture. You need to be careful in areas of unnaturally high ultraviolet radiation due to the effects that it may have on the human mind and body. The peak areas in society for these ultraviolet effects appears to occur around glass covered buildings. When around such buildings, you should wear a hat, cover up, and pass through the areas of high ultraviolet radiation quickly.

In areas around tall glass covered buildings, the sky is very different. If you look up at certain times of the day, you may actually see two or more Sun's in the sky! You will see the real Sun and one or more reflected Sun's. This increases the ground based radiation levels and the effect on human health is not fully understood yet. Until it is, it pays to exercise caution around it. The effect is called "The Multiple-Sun Effect".

This effect was headline news in 2010 and the press called it the "Las Vegas Death Ray" due to a curved, mirrored, glass covered hotel in Las Vegas exhibiting the problem. The radiation levels on the ground were getting so high that the plastic drinking cups were melting! One can only wonder what extended exposure to the human mind and body would cause. The effect of focusing sunlight with mirrors was documented by Archimedes a long time ago as the "Archimedes Death Ray" and its purpose was for setting invading ships on fire.

The following pages show some of the solar radiation effects that you should be aware of:

The "Multiple-Sun" Effect

Building glass can create the "Multiple-Sun" effect.

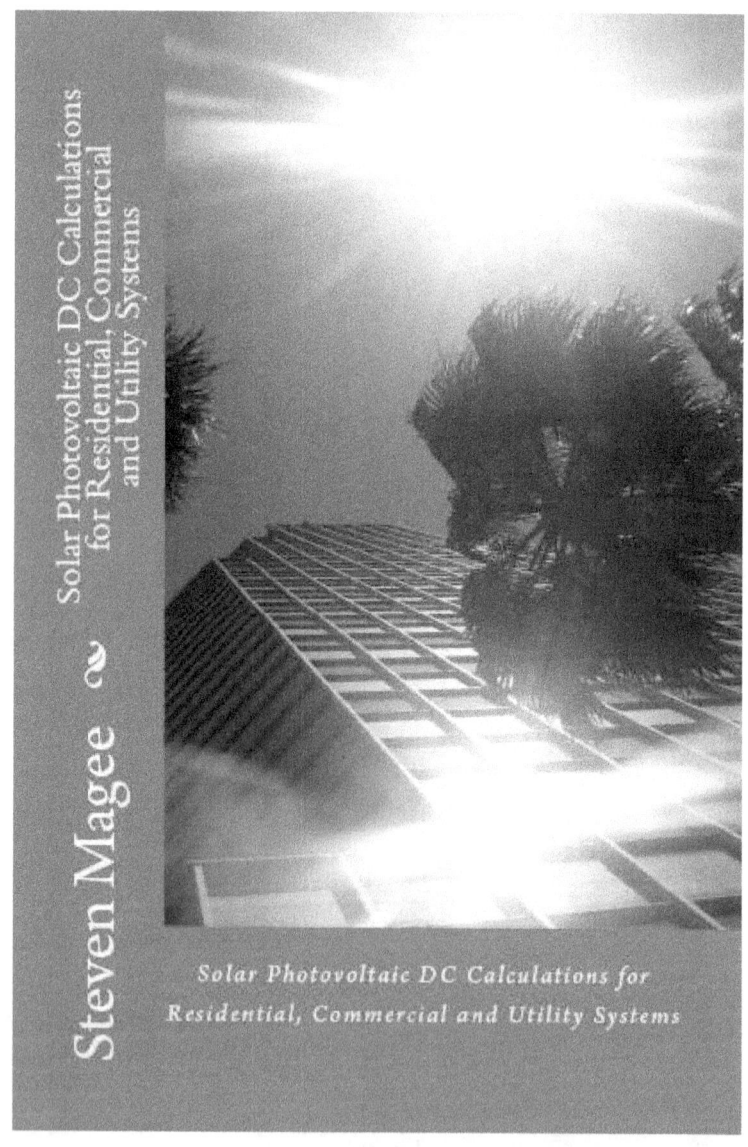

The "Multiple-Shadow" Effect

The "Multiple-Shadow" effect accompanies the "Multiple-Sun" effect. The bright area on the right is higher in solar radiation power than Space!

"Archimedes Death Ray" Effect

Curved buildings can create the "Archimedes Death Ray".

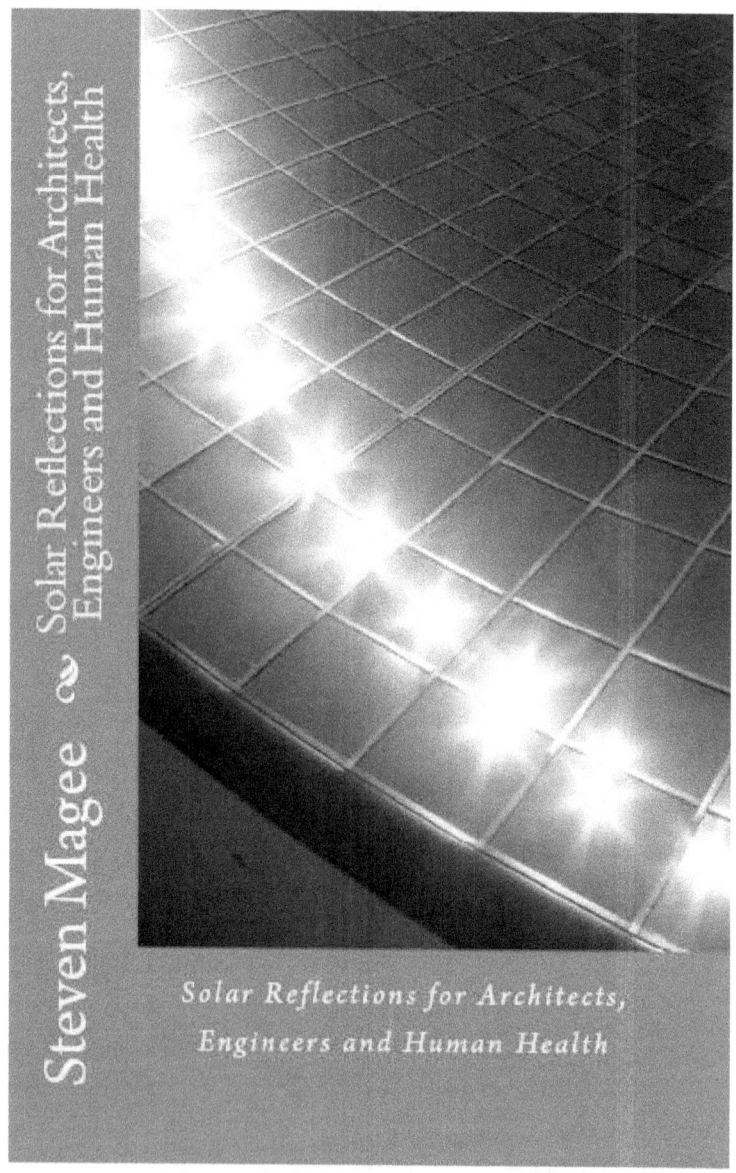

Steven Magee ∾ Solar Reflections for Architects, Engineers and Human Health

Solar Reflections for Architects, Engineers and Human Health

Toxic Health © Steven Magee

"Multiple-Sun" Effect in Cars

The "Multiple-Sun" effect occurs in cars.

Possible Interference Cloud Formation

Holes in the clouds may cause filtering, interference effects, and high solar radiation cycling on the human mind and body.

Colors in Clouds

Colors in clouds may be solar radiation interference effects.

So you are worried about artificial lighting and are thinking that you can fix it by using full spectrum lighting products? Think again! While full spectrum lighting products sound appealing, the truth is that there is no such thing as full spectrum artificial lighting. It is a marketing ploy.

What full spectrum really means is that the light is as close to the Sun's spectrum as can be possibly made using current technology. Unfortunately, it is not sunlight and never will be.

All types of artificial lighting have the possibility of making you ill. Artificial lighting should be avoided if your health is important to you.

If you are going to have artificial lighting in your environment, then it should have a plant in front of it so that the light becomes modified by the plant. This is shown on the next page.

Toxic Health © Steven Magee

Light Modification by Plants

Here is the "Star of Bethlehem" as produced by a halogen lamp and a plant.

Toxic Health © Steven Magee

Color temperatures can be used to specify light sources. Here is a list of the color temperatures in Kelvin of modern light sources, as listed on Wikipedia:

- 1,700K Match flame.

- 1,850K Candle flame, sunset/sunrise.

- 2,700–3,300K Incandescent light bulb.

- 3,350K Studio "CP" light.

- 3,400K Studio lamps, photofloods, etc.

- 4,100K Moonlight, xenon arc lamp.

- 5,000K Horizon daylight.

- 5,500–6,000K Vertical daylight, electronic flash.

- 6,500K Daylight, overcast.

- 9,300K CRT screen.

As can be seen, the color temperature varies between the different sources and also the different times of the day.

The Color Rendering Index, or CRI for short, is similar to the color temperature. Wikipedia says the *"Color rendering index, or CRI, is a measure of the quality of color light, devised by the International Commission on Illumination (CIE). It generally ranges from zero for a source like a low-pressure sodium vapor lamp, which is monochromatic, to one hundred, for a source like an incandescent light bulb, which emits essentially blackbody radiation. It is related to color temperature, in that the CRI measures for a pair of light sources can only be compared if they have the same color temperature. A standard "cool white" fluorescent lamp will have a CRI near 62."*

The color temperature and CRI do not give the full picture. You also need to be aware of the radiation spectrum. Unfortunately, most gas discharge lamps have a spiked radiation spectrum that does not occur in nature. Due to this, you should avoid any artificial lighting that is created from gas discharge sources, such as mercury vapor, fluorescent, sodium, neon, and so on.

Dr. John Nash Ott found that he could change the gender of plants and animals simply by changing the color temperature of the artificial lights that they were exposed to! A very interesting effect of artificial lighting and it is a good reason to ensure that you have the correct lighting products in your home and office, and particularly around babies and developing children.

Mercury based lighting mystifies me. We know that mercury is toxic to humans. So why would we make lighting products with it? Dr. John Nash Ott extensively demonstrated in his books that many mercury lighting products appear to be harmful to human health.

The next page shows how the florescent (mercury) and tungsten (traditional) light bulb spectrums compare.

Florescent Spectrum

Note that the spectral lines are not continuous, but rather broken up. This is typical of gas discharge lighting. It does not occur in nature.

Tungsten Spectrum

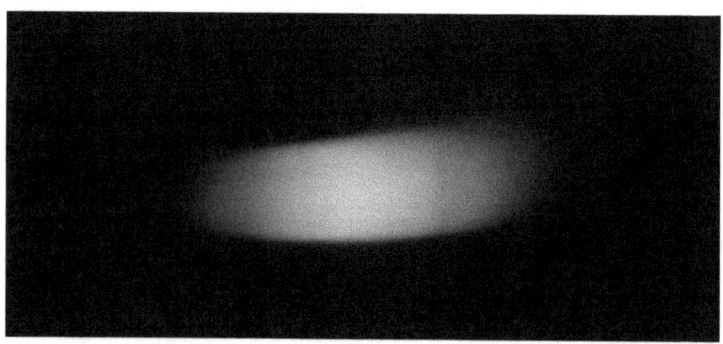

A smooth continuous spectrum that is typical of what nature produces.

I would recommend that you avoid the use of the new lighting that has been developed, such as gas discharge and light emitting diode (LED) lighting. These have been developed in order to use less energy at the expense of the quality of the light. They are typically not comparable to natural sources of light and they may make you ill in the long term.

All artificial lighting should be generated by heat. This is how the Sun generates light. Unfortunately, there are no man-made sources of lighting that can generate the same temperature as the Sun. Halogen filament lighting is about as close as it gets.

Television and computer displays of all types are sources of artificial light. You should be wary of your exposure to these as they may be able to impact your health.

The recent adoption of large screen televisions may bring with it an increase in human health problems in the future. People watching three dimensional images frequently may be an issue in the long term. Both of these could possibly be like a ticking time bomb. It is recommended that if you have a display in your environment that you keep it as small as possible. You may want to experiment with the brightness and contrast controls to get it to emit the lowest amount of light and still be comfortable to use. It is advised that your screen should not dominate your field of view.

Use your display in an environment that has good lighting in it and plenty of plants. Your display should not be the brightest thing in your environment.

So what is a healthy level of lighting? If we take a look at the forest environment, then the answer is obvious. Keep daytime lighting levels equivalent to outdoor shade values and use plants in front of artificial lights to create light filtering and interference. Use natural plants in front of your windows to create light filtering and interference. If indoors, you should sit facing the window during the daytime so that your eyes can sense the changing levels of daylight. It is preferable for your windows to be at eye level when seated so that you can see the outdoors through them.

A simple way of gauging the indoor daytime light environment for the human is to do a light test. Turn off your indoor lighting in the middle of the day. Note how bright the surroundings are. Now turn on your indoor lights and see if it is brighter. If the indoor environment is brighter then it means that you need to have more natural light coming in to your daytime areas. You can do this by adding more windows or skylights.

You should be aiming to illuminate your indoor daytime environment with natural outdoor light, not electrical lighting products. This light should be full spectrum natural light that the intensity can be controlled with window shades. Working in daytime environments that are illuminated with artificial lighting products is undesirable for human health.

If you work in a daytime indoor environment, then the lighting should mimic what nature does. It should have a natural daytime spectrum of light that matches outdoor daylight. This would be achieved with full spectrum filament lights that have the correct amount of blue and ultraviolet light in their spectrums to mimic outdoor daylight. Your indoor lighting level should be approximately 1,000 lux (Lux is a measurement of brightness of light).

From 10:00 to 14:00 there should be an additional set of lights that is turned on that increases the brightness of the office environment, to mimic the peak in daylight that occurs outdoors. The indoor environment during this time should have an illumination level of approximately 2,000 lux. You can easily achieve this in your office environment by simply having a desk lamp that you switch on during that time to increase the light illumination that you are exposed to. You should be using full spectrum filament light bulbs of the correct spectral emissions for this exposure.

You should make sure that you go outdoors for an hour at solar noon and sit in the shade of trees. Do not wear any sunglasses, glasses, contacts, make-up, nor sunscreen for this exposure. You need this exposure daily to keep up the solar cycle in the human mind and body. Without it, you may start to get fatigued as the day goes on. Daily outdoor exposure to sunlight is very important if you have an indoor occupation.

If you do not get the correct light exposures in the day, then your sleep cycle may kick in. The human mind and body when kept in an indoor environment of low lux light will not realize that it is daytime, as it cannot sense the increasing levels of daylight that the genetics are accustomed to. As such, by late morning your body may start sending a signal for you to sleep!

If you can, during any of your daily breaks, you should try and go outdoors to get natural daylight. You will also be getting fresh air and pollen exposure, which are also necessary for good health.

The recommended cycle for indoor daytime lighting is shown on the next page.

Indoor Daytime Lighting Cycle for Human Health

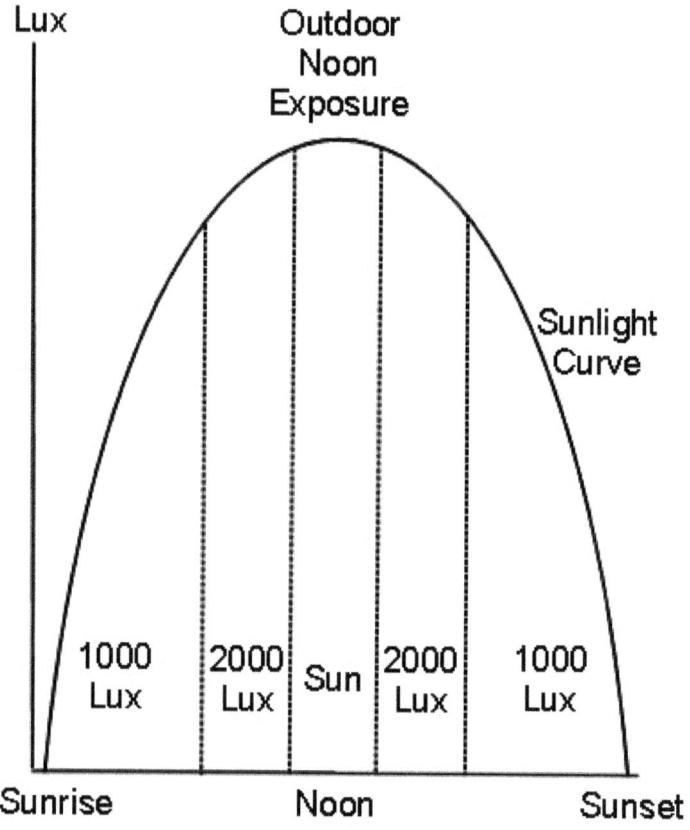

Nighttime lighting is very different from daytime lighting. You want to be using products that have minimal blue light in them. Blue light exposure is well known to cause insomnia. If you install lighting products that have too much blue light in their spectrums, then you may enter into a life of insomnia and not realize that it is your light bulbs that are causing it! Insomnia rapidly leads to fatigue and onto depression. These daytime lighting products are commonly sold as "Daylight" or "Full Spectrum" light bulbs and should not be used in nighttime applications.

You should stick to the tried and tested filament light bulbs for your nighttime exposures. Avoid the compact florescent and LED bulbs as some of these are well known for their excessive blue light content. Keep your lights low, as bright light can also trigger insomnia.

Most people do not actually realize it, but they are polluting the interior of their homes with nighttime electric lighting. This pollution has become quite severe in the last few decades with the adoption of compact florescent lights (CFL) and light emitting diode (LED) products. These products typically have unnatural spectrums of light and can have a wide range of electromagnetic interference emissions from them. Some of them give out too much blue light and this may induce insomnia and macular degeneration of the eye. They can turn the home wiring into a radio transmitter which may lead to Electromagnetic Hypersensitivity in the human.

I currently advise people to use filament bulbs. I presently use conventional filament light bulbs for nighttime lighting at my home. I keep the lighting low and just sufficient for what I am doing.

Low voltage halogen lighting products should be avoided due to the emissions from them. They may have high amounts of man-made ultraviolet light, some create dirty electricity, and electric and magnetic fields. Man-made ultraviolet light is known for its ability to cause skin and eye problems and ultraviolet light is not present during the nighttime in nature. You will not find any electronic lamp dimmers in my

Toxic Health © Steven Magee

home, as they are a product that you should avoid using. Lamp dimmers can create dirty electricity, electric and magnetic fields.

You should also be using the correct voltage light bulb. In the USA these are sold as either 120 volt or 130 volt light bulbs. You should be using the 120 volt versions, as they are far more efficient at producing light. The 130 volt versions should only be used if your light bulbs are frequently breaking within a few days of installing them. If you use 130 volt light bulbs when they are not needed, your light bulbs will last a very long time, but will give out a poor quality of light.

You should be aware that the many sources of artificial lighting can affect your mental and physical health. You should be choosing your daytime artificial lighting products based on the proven health benefits of "Full Spectrum" light bulbs that are comparable to outdoor daylight. Health benefits have been reported by many gardeners who use these products to grow their plants indoors during the winter months. Nighttime artificial lighting products are different to daytime products and should be used in your home for good sleep patterns.

Nighttime over-illumination is a problem in the modern world and it may be able to affect your health. Keep it as low as possible during the nighttime and only increase lighting levels if you feel that you need more light in your environment. You should think candles, not necessarily use candles, but rather the illumination level that candles create. There is a reason why candles are considered romantic and it is likely related to the low level of light that they create.

If you have your environment too bright during the nighttime, then you may upset the circadian rhythm that governs your sleep cycles. Keep lighting as low as possible during the nighttime. You should also keep your skin covered as much as possible to prevent it from absorbing the artificial light.

You should be wary of computer monitors and televisions, as their light can be very unnatural and may induce a wide range of health problems into you. The most common problem is insomnia and this can be reduced by adjusting the blue color on the monitor lower and minimal brightness. Using televisions and computers after dark is not advisable and may adversely affect your sleep.

During the daytime, you should use your computer next to a shady full spectrum window to dilute the artificial light from the monitor with natural daylight. If you work in an office where you cannot see the outdoors, then you should place a full spectrum diffused light behind your monitor with plants to give you a more natural light exposure to the eyes and skin.

The correct daytime alignment of a computer monitor is shown in the next picture.

It is likely that daytime office environments would be healthier if the ceiling was painted sky blue and the walls had green nature landscape scenes on them. Clearly, the office staff sitting facing shady full spectrum windows is already proven for its beneficial health effects and has been so for many decades. You should be aiming to keep your environment as natural as possible for good human health. Natural potted plants can assist in this process in the office environment.

A spectrograph can be used to assess the quality of light in your environment and you can buy affordable spectrographs from scientific education suppliers and astronomical shops. You can easily build a simple spectrograph out of a cardboard box and a compact disk to enable you to assess the different types of lighting products in your environment. I built mine in just ten minutes! This is shown on the following pages.

Computer Screen Alignment

The correct alignment of a computer screen to the shaded full spectrum ultraviolet transmitting acrylic window. You should try and ensure that you have a natural view behind a computer monitor during the daytime.

Spectrograph Design

Here is the design of a cereal box spectrograph using a standard compact disk, from:
http://www.cs.cmu.edu/~zhuxj/astro/html/spectrometer.html

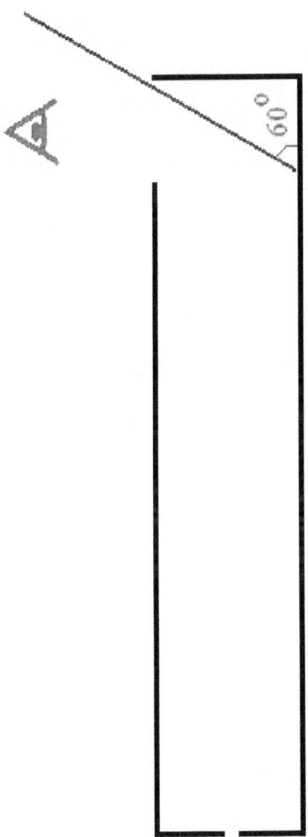

Spectrograph

Here is the cereal box spectrograph.

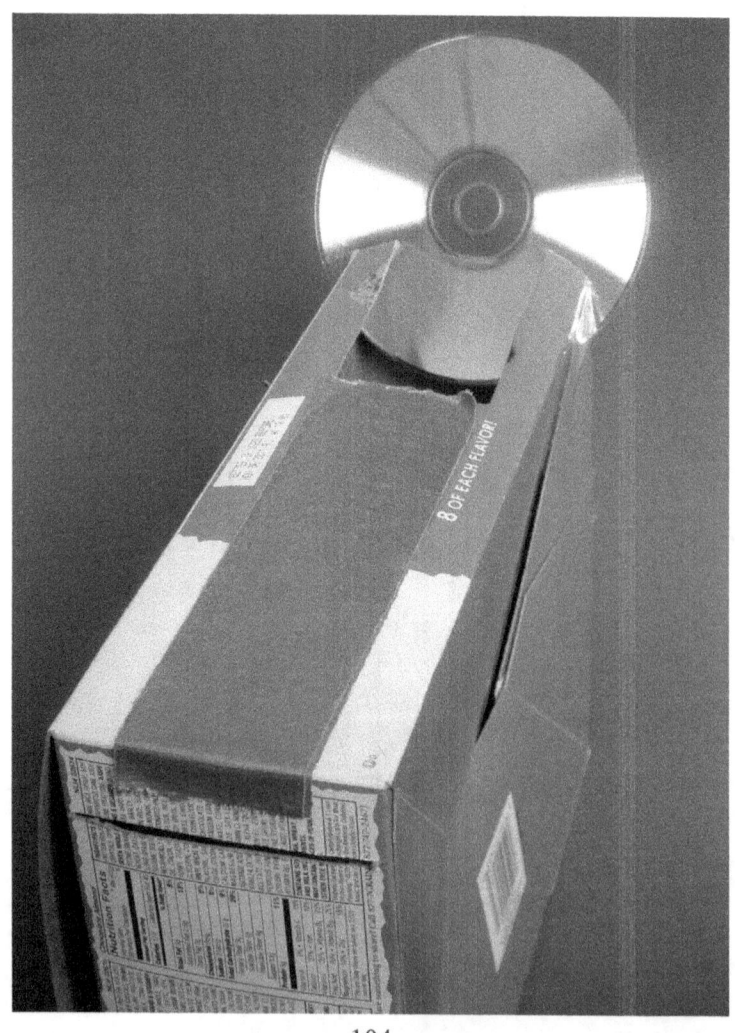

Spectrograph in Operation

A spectrum of a florescent light produced by the cereal box spectrograph. Note the bands of distinct colors of light. These do not occur in light produced by nature.

Incorrect radiation levels may be able to affect your sex drive and it may be proven in the future that human sex drive is governed more by radiation types and levels than any other factor, even more so than hormones! Generally, a feeling of contentment replaces sexual desire in natural radiation environments.

We are constantly walking around in an energy field of broad spectrum solar radiation that originated at the largest nuclear reactor in the solar system, called the Sun. It is important that this energy level be kept low for human health. The trees and plants, also known as nature, provide this function and aid human health.

You should avoid watching the sunrises and sunsets regularly due to the filtered nature of the solar radiation. It is this filtering that generates the amazing colors. Unfortunately, staring at the Sun during this time appears to be bad for human health. It may have the potential to make you ill through solar radiation induced disease if it becomes a regular habit. You should be wary of the orange and red colors that occur during this time, as they may be a product of atmospheric pollution.

General exposure to the direct view of the Sun delivers a lot of energy to your mind and body and this can be felt as heat and also sensed by the eyes as brightness and you may need to wear sunglasses due to this. There are no doubts that the Sun is a carcinogen in the wrong situation and it is wise to avoid direct views of it in a developed environment.

Glass rooms, such as conservatories, should be avoided. They are generally full of reflections and these boost the radiation levels inside them. If you have one of these rooms, you would be wise to fill it with plant life in order to reduce the solar radiation levels inside it.

East, equatorial (south in northern hemisphere and north in southern hemisphere) and west facing windows let in a lot of direct solar radiation. You should not spend time too close to windows in this orientation. Window shades and coverings are recommended. Plants should be placed next to windows like this. Desks should not be placed under

windows that have direct sunlight as you will get overheated and fatigued. Longer term, you may develop radiation sickness.

As for your eyes, ultraviolet (UV) blocking sunglasses should be worn when the solar radiation levels are unnaturally high and these should be of an appropriate level of neutral density optical material. Mirrored, colored or polarized lenses should be avoided due to the modification of the solar radiation that takes place with these. Solar and artificial radiation viewed through glasses and contact lenses may be able to impact your health and you should only wear them as needed. You should view the light that your eyes receive as a nutrient and you want to keep it as natural as possible.

A picture of the Sun through a pair of tri-focal glasses is shown on the next page. Bi-focal and tri-focal glasses may be a particular issue for solar radiation transmission to the eye.

Toxic Health © Steven Magee

Sunlight Through Tri-focal Glasses

The Sun appears to have magnification, filtering, and interference effects when viewed through tri-focal glasses.

Anything unnatural that filters the broad spectrum of solar radiation will create an artificial and possibly toxic environment for humans. Unnaturally filtering sunlight may cause it to create electromagnetic interference (EMI) effects in the human body. We will discuss the effects of EMI later.

Glass coatings modify the solar radiation spectrum on both the outside and inside of the glass. Many of these coatings cannot be seen by the human eye and the glass will appear to be transparent to optical light. The glass may be highly reflective to other wavelengths such as ultraviolet (UV), infrared (IR), microwave, radio, and so on.

The following pictures show the difference between outdoor light and indoor light. The first picture was taken outside looking at the reflection of the metal plate on the bench. The second picture was taken from inside the home looking through a coated double glazed window and mesh screen. As can be seen, the white outdoor light changes to yellow with many rainbow colored spikes when viewed from inside the home.

Outside Light

The reflected white sunlight from the bench, as photographed outdoors. Note the wisps of light.

Inside Light

This picture was taken from inside the home through coated
double glazed glass and a mesh screen. Note the yellow light
and the rainbow effects in the spikes.

The atmosphere when mixed with pollution is just like a window coating. If you fill the atmosphere with toxins, then you really cannot be surprised if the solar radiation transmission through it becomes toxic to humans.

The next picture shows the Sun as viewed from the window of an airplane. As you can see, the Sun is white, but the reflection from the ocean is orange! The filtering of the sunlight by the polluted atmosphere has changed the color of the sunlight to orange.

The following picture shows the pollution that can be found hanging over Los Angeles, California. This will filter the sunlight during the day and the astronomical light during the night. It is not a good idea to live in large cities such as this if your health is important to you.

The Sun as Viewed from an Airplane.

This picture was taken from an airplane window at cruising altitude in the Pacific ocean near to Hawaii. Note the white Sun and orange reflection below.

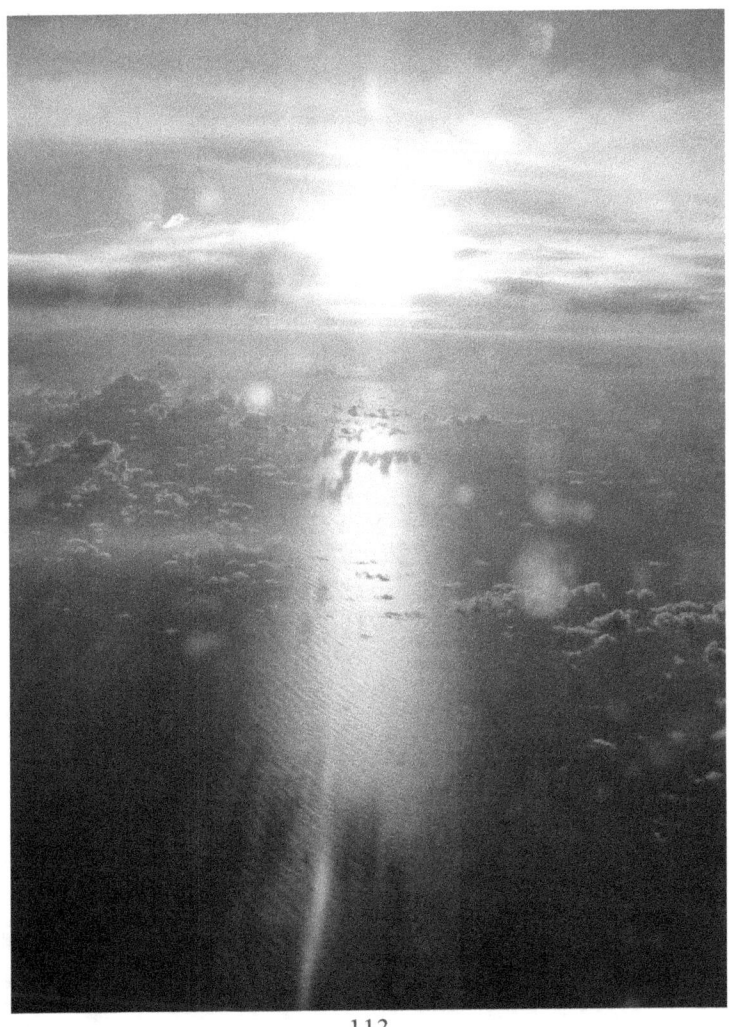

City Pollution

The band of atmospheric pollution hanging over Los Angeles, California, as viewed from the Griffith Observatory. Pollution will unnaturally filter light.

This appears to be the current understanding of solar radiation power levels on the human mind and body:

Too Low: Sunlight deficiency, developmental problems, deformities in babies, bone deformity in the young, rickets, system deficiencies, low vitamin D, low vitamin B12, high cholesterol, muscle weakness, legs may feel heavy, difficulty moving, aches and pains, hunger, vomiting, nausea, diarrhea, obesity, anxiety, stress, mental issues, fatigue, depression symptoms, headaches, moodiness, eye issues, Attention Deficit Disorder (ADD), Autism, general illness, shorter or longer life span (reduced aging effects from sunlight exposure may lengthen the lifespan, whereas the sickness effects of the deficiencies may shorten it).

Low: Extended lifespan from reduced solar radiation aging effects.

Normal: Unlimited energy during the day. Good sleep patterns. Excellent health. Clear thinking. Normal development. Normal life span.

Above Normal: Extended life span from increased radiation exposure, system under stress, general illness.

High: Accelerated development, may have reduced height as an adult, accelerated aging, going gray prematurely, hypochondriac symptoms, sleep problems, anxiety, stress, eye issues, mental issues, fatigue, depression, random aches and pains, itchy skin, hot skin, system overload, immune system compromised, cold sores, intestinal problems.

Too High: In addition to above: Deformities in babies, bone deformity in the young, frequent illness, onset of disease, most likely premature death.

Extreme: In addition to above: Rapid onset of disease, major eye issues, premature death.

Unnatural sources of radiation (such as mercury lamps) may change the speed of progression of these problems and will most likely speed it up.

Constantly changing between the different levels (high cycling) may be able to induce mental instability or depression.

Changing from low solar radiation exposure to high during a day may cause an intoxication effect to occur. You may feel hungover the next day if you are sunlight deficient.

It is well known that life expectancy is modified according to radiation exposure. The next graph shows what I have been able to ascertain about how this occurs.

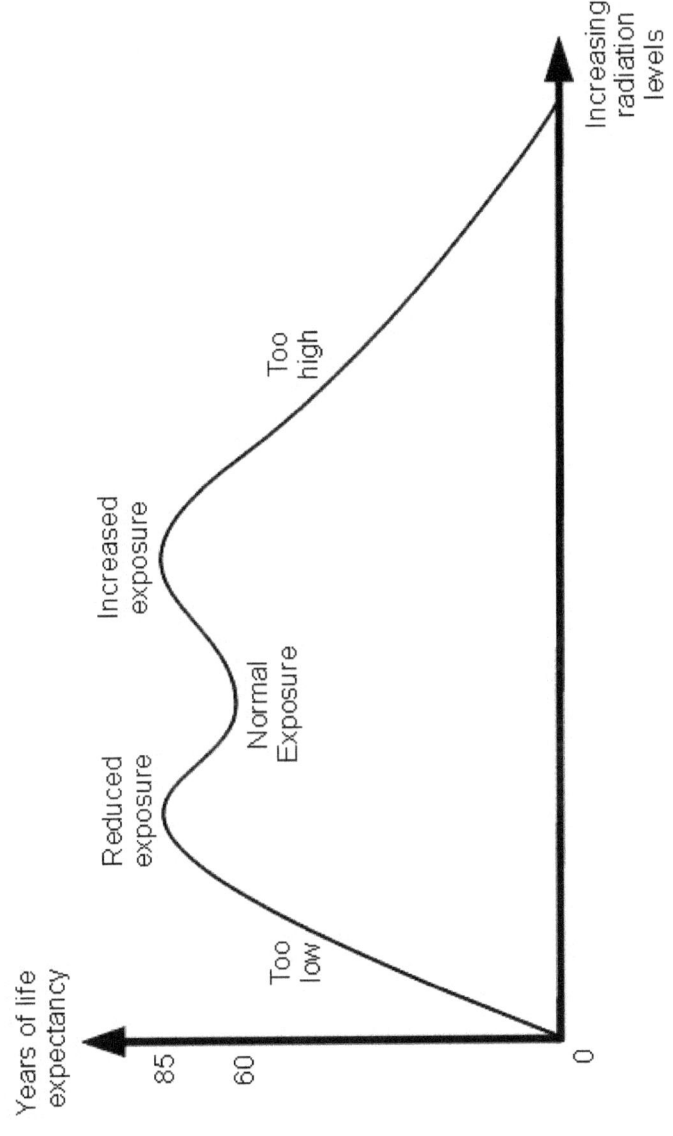

Life Expectancy Radiation Exposures

The definition of a normal level of solar radiation for humans is a forested environment in the tropics that has a tree canopy. This is due to the "Tree Canopy Light Interference" effect.

The human skin is referred to by many as the largest organ of the human body. As the largest organ, it also has the largest task in the body. It is your suit of armor against the environment and for it to work well requires attention on your part.

The human skin is sensitive to radiation. Expose it to solar radiation and it will start to react to it and make changes to the human mind and body. The levels of radiation of all types needs to be controlled to natural levels in order for the changes that they create to be beneficial to humans.

The use of sunscreens are not recommended. Sunscreens act like window coatings and modify the solar radiation received by the body. There is much talk about sunscreen being potentially poisonous to the human body. Instead, use natural methods such as shade, an umbrella, a wide brimmed hat, and white clothing to protect yourself from excessive Sun exposure. It is interesting to note that human clothing styles changed significantly over the last century and prior to this it was normal to cover up the human body when in sunlight. Exposing lots of skin to the direct view of the Sun is a relatively new trend in humans, as is sunbathing.

Many traditional cultures have understood the need to cover up the skin when in direct sunlight and, in men, to grow beards. Keeping hair to its natural length in all parts of the body appears to be a protector against radiation. Of interest is that hair may do this through the use of solar radiation interference as well as blocking the radiation.

If your eyes or body get too much Sun exposure and start to exhibit problem(s), you should retreat indoors and allow the problem(s) to clear up. You should still get daily outdoor exposure, but stay in the shade and keep it to about an hour until you fully recover. You will need to be careful that you do not go into sunlight withdrawal when recovering from Sun damage.

The human mind and body has a very advanced photosynthesis mechanism that keeps it functioning well. It is important that the human mind and body is exposed daily to the natural light that occurs in nature and this is found under the tree canopy in a green natural environment. The UK has found this out the hard way with 20% of the children tested showing signs of rickets in 2010!

Clear ultra-violet (UV) transmitting acrylic window products are available and are commonly used by zoo's to prevent the animals becoming vitamin D deficient. It is recommended that you have these products installed where you spend the bulk of your daytime activities. This is especially important around developing children, as UV is known to be important in the correct development of children. Products that are specifically marketed for this purpose are "Monkey Shine" Solarcryl SUVT and LuciteLux Utran UVT. These are products that are commonly used in tanning beds and they have a high UV light transmission. You can easily obtain these products from tanning bed manufacturers and suppliers.

I have installed this in my office and my kitchen where I spend most of my day. My initial findings are that it has helped improve the final health problem that I am trying to eliminate, which is occasional fatigue. If you have developing babies and children, then you should install this in areas where they spend the bulk of their daytime. Full spectrum windows are particularly important for them. You do not need to install this in areas where you spend your evening and nighttime, such as bedrooms and bathrooms.

You should be aware that you can get sunburned through these products and that many things, such as plastics, may suffer from ultraviolet degradation. It is preferable to install UV transmitting glazing in areas that are shaded, such as the side of your home that faces the pole. In sunny locations, you should ensure that your window shades and coverings can sufficiently reduce the sunlight levels to prevent you from getting sunburn!

Dr. John Nash Ott installed UV transmitting plastic windows in his home. This was due to noticing that his plants were not growing correctly indoors behind the glass windows. The UV transmitting products that he used improved the growth patterns. He also said that it improved his own health. He reported having better eyesight, thicker hair, far fewer incidences of colds and the flu, and excellent health after installing it.

There is one last thing that we need to look into and that is the question of "What is nighttime?". One answer to this question that I have heard is that it is an absence of daylight. Having given it some thought and become aware of effects that are taking place in plants during the nighttime, I now know this not to be entirely correct.

Nighttime appears to be a heavily filtered and interference form of daytime. There is some daylight still present during the night, it is just that our human eyes are not able to detect it. Animals that have night vision have evolved with eyes that are able to function in this much lower level of daylight. Illumination by the stars becomes prevalent, each of which is a nuclear reactor. The cycles of the moon and planets come into play, as do comets and shooting stars. Nighttime also has a very different radio frequency environment due to the lack of ionization of the atmosphere from solar radiation absorption.

On the way to nighttime we pass through the period known as sunset. This period marks a distinct change that lasts approximately two hours where great changes in the lighting levels and types of radiation occur. At sunset as the Sun is coming down to the horizon, the light becomes an interference type of light due to crossing the horizon and also by being heavily filtered by the atmosphere. The same effect happens at sunrise. Sunrise is different from sunset due to the air being cooler. As such, less interference and filtering effects take place during sunrise.

The diagram on the next page shows the cycles of light over one day. The following diagram shows the solar radiation daytime and nighttime effects that take place. The last diagram shows the interference effects that may occur during a solar eclipse by the Moon.

Moon Interference with Earth

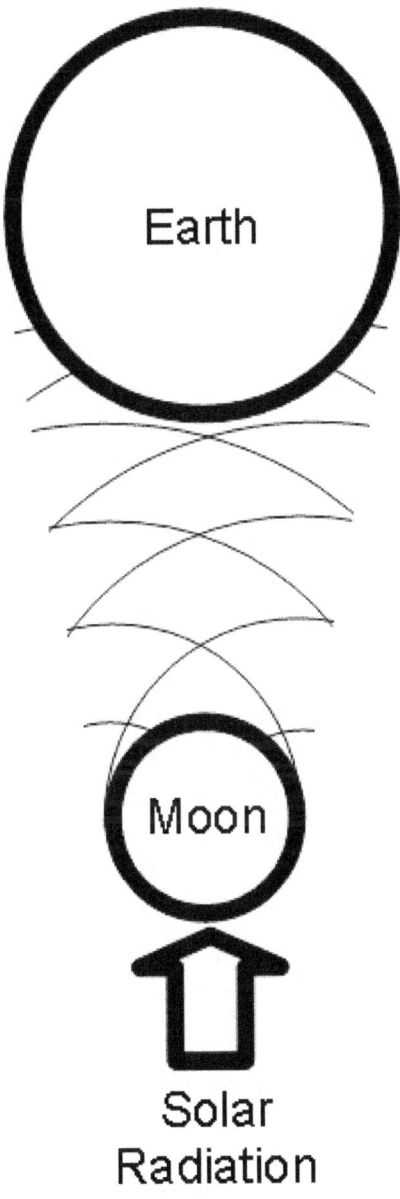

Light in the human environment is an extensive subject that has many more facets than what we can cover in this chapter. As such, more information on light in the human environment can be found in my book on the subject, called "Toxic Light".

"Health and Light" by Dr. John Nash Ott is also recommended for further reading on this subject.

The human health advantages of effective Sun exposure are documented in the following books:

- "Sunlight" by Zane R. Kime MD MS.

- "The Healing Sun: Sunlight and Health in the 21st Century" by Richard Hobday PhD.

- "Light: Medicine of the Future" by Jacob Liberman OD PhD.

- "The UV Advantage" by Michael F Holick PhD MD and Mark Jenkins.

Trees are extensively documented for their health and healing powers on the human mind and body and the following books are recommended reading:

- "The Healing Power of Forests: The Philosophy Behind Restoring Earth's Balance with Native Trees." by Akira Miyawaki and Elgene O. Box.

- "The Healing Power of Trees: Spiritual Journeys Through the Celtic Calendar." by Sharlyn Hidalgo.

"Eating the Sun: How Plants Power the Planet" by Oliver Martin explores the solar functions of plants further.

"Only a full spectrum of natural light could promote full health in plants, animals, and humans."

Dr. John Nash Ott

Toxic Health © Steven Magee

<u>Sleep</u>

One of the things that has disappeared for many people is their quality of sleep. I can associate with this as I was plagued with insomnia for many years that I eventually traced to side effects of medications, artificial lighting products and electromagnetic interference exposures. How wonderful it was to get great sleep patterns back!

Most biological damage appears to occur during sleep. Sleep is the regeneration process of the mind and body and for it to work well requires the natural environmental conditions that humans evolved in.

You should pay close attention to your bedroom environment. You should be concerned when you open your eyes in the middle of the night and can see things. Your bedroom should be completely dark while you sleep. You should not be able to see anything!

Things that should not be in your bedroom are:

- Night lights.
- LED clocks.
- Cell phones.
- Wireless products.
- Electricity.
- Products that glow.

Your bedroom is where you go to biologically regenerate. It must be completely dark for this process to work well. It is undesirable to have electricity in the room and electrical products as they may interfere with the regeneration process. If you have light coming into the room, then you should purchase blackout blinds to prevent it. You should regard your

126

bedroom as a refuge of darkness where you recharge for the next day of light. Simply Yin and Yang.

One of the techniques that I developed when recovering my health was rotational sleeping. I developed this technique when I became aware that there are now biological hotspots of wireless radiation in homes today. The technique revolves around making sure that you do not sleep in the same position each night. The simplest form of the technique is to move your pillow to the opposite end of the bed from the previous night, so that you rotate 180 degrees each night. I prefer to sleep in a four position rotation cycle and this works well in large beds. I follow this pattern in a large bed:

1. **Left side of bed.**
2. **Rotate 180 degrees.**
3. **Right side of bed.**
4. **Rotate 180 degrees.**

This means that if there is a biological hotspot where your head rests, then it will only be subjected to that hotspot one night in every four. You should pay attention to how you feel when you wake up each day and if one of the positions is constantly making you fatigued in the morning, you should consider moving your bed to a different location.

A useful technique for assessing the quality of the environment in your bedrooms is the "Goldilocks" test. If you have multiple bedrooms, then spend a week sleeping in each bedroom and see how you feel. The bedroom that you wake up feeling really refreshed in is the one where you should sleep.

If there is a high powered transmitter near to your home, then you should align your bed so that it presents the least bodily area to the transmitter. It is preferable to have your feet pointing toward the transmitter and your head pointing away from it.

This configuration will ensure the least irradiation of the brain occurs, as it will be shielded by the body.

If you are raising babies and children, I recommend that you sleep in their rooms for a week and see how you feel. If you are not waking up refreshed, then it is likely that they are not waking up refreshed either. If this is the case, you should consider moving them into another room or have an expert come in to assess what the problem is in the bedroom. I recommend that parents of Autistic children change the bedroom that their Autistic child sleeps in to see if it improves their health.

Sleeping on the floor is known for its health benefits and many people do it. The radio frequency fields are very low at the ground and I have found that it improved my health for several months after being subjected to a high powered pulsed radio frequency field from the utility meter. You should make sure that the floor that you are sleeping on does not have stray voltage or any electrical cables running through it. I eventually had to stop sleeping on my floor due to seasonal stray voltage/current/frequency detrimental health effects that showed up as the voltage on the floor increased. I suspect that this sleeping on the floor technique may be beneficial to some Autistic children.

Metal bed frames with metal mattresses are undesirable in a wireless radiation society. The metal coil mattress is an antenna system that will have a wide range of electromagnetic energy flowing on it. Metal can be radioactive if it was contaminated during its manufacture. Occasionally, an X-ray machine will be melted down during the metal recycling process and contaminate the entire batch of metal. Metal also disturbs the natural magnetic field of the Earth and this is undesirable for the cellular regeneration processes. Melanoma and breast cancer are suspected to be linked to sleeping on metal coil mattresses.

Wooden bed frames with natural foam mattresses are recommended. A low wooden bed frame that keeps you about one foot above the floor appears to be the ideal height to avoid stray voltage/current/frequency exposures that may be on the concrete floor and for reducing exposure to radio frequencies. If you have electrical wiring running under the wooden floor that your bed is on, then it is recommended to have the fields of that wiring assessed and to ensure that the mattress is high enough off the floor to avoid those fields. Keep the bed out of the electrical wiring fields that may be in the walls by keeping it a few feet away from the wall or by turning off the bedroom electrical circuit during the night.

Nature defines the human sleep environment as dark with low radiation levels and you should ensure that during the nighttime that you are sleeping in this environment.

"In order for the light to shine so brightly, the darkness must be present."

Francis Bacon

Radiation

"It is clear that radiation produces the electrical current which operates adaptively the organism as a whole, producing memory, reason, imagination, emotion, the special senses, secretions, muscular action, the response to infection, normal growth, and the growth of benign tumors and cancers, all of which are governed adaptively by the electric charges that are generated by the short wave or ionizing radiation in protoplasm."

Dr. George Crile

Most people associate radiation with nuclear bombs, nuclear power plants and X-ray machines. This is a very blinkered view and we will show you how extensive radiation in the human environment is and how critical it is for human health.

The modern human has created a radiation environment that has never existed before in all of human history and it keeps on adding to it every year. This is an issue as most of the sources of man-made radiation are not yet fully understood. As a radiation society, we are running before we have even learned to crawl!

The radiation environment started to significantly change at the start of the Industrial Revolution when the steam engines started to fill the atmosphere with water vapor, wood and coal burning emissions. This later progressed onto gas and oil burning in the late 1800's as the wood and coal became harder to source. How would this affect the radiation environment? Well, by cutting down the trees, the tree canopy was destroyed which caused the solar radiation levels to significantly increase!

The tree canopy typically reduces the solar radiation power levels between 10 and 30 times less through absorption and modification of the solar radiation. This is important to human health as the mind and body does not function well in a direct view of the Sun and may eventually get ill.

Toxic Health © Steven Magee

It is somewhat ironic that during the settling of the USA, that the government required many of the settlers to clear the land that was given to them! Poor health born out of greatly increased solar radiation levels may have followed this action.

As for the emissions into the atmosphere, this has changed the solar radiation transmission from Space to the ground. The solar radiation all around the world is now significantly different from what it was just a few hundred years ago. As the emissions continue into the atmosphere, the solar radiation will become changed so much that many people will start to become ill with radiation sickness. In some parts of the world, it is likely that this is already happening.

But solar radiation is just a small part of the story. The human radiation environment has many aspects to it:

- Solar radiation.
- Environmental radiation.
- Radio waves.
- Microwaves.
- Electrical and electronic radiation.

Environmental radiation can come from many sources:

- Cosmic radiation.
- Electrical storms.
- Replacing nature with modern development significantly raises the levels of many types of radiation.
- Mining activities bring radioactive minerals to the surface which will increase the background radiation levels.
- Fall out from nuclear bombs and power plant disasters.

131

- Living close to a nuclear power station.
- Living close to a power generation plant.
- Living at altitude.
- Living near large bodies of water.
- Living in snowy climates.
- Living close to a military base.
- Living close to an airport or port.
- Living close to any type of broadcast antenna.
- Living close to power poles and lines.
- Living close to tall structures.

Man-made electrical and electronic radiation did not exist until the 1700's when scientists started to discover the various forms of it. We have progressed extremely quickly from a new discovery to the many forms of it that are now present in modern society and this seems to have happened with little thought to the consequences to human health.

We now live in a society that is bombarded by electrical, electronic and wireless radiation. There is no place in the world that it does not reach with the prolific adoption of satellite and radio communications. Future historians will likely document this as one of the most foolish things that humanity ever did.

The electrical, electronic and wireless interference is commonly called:

- Electromagnetic Interference (EMI).
- Radio Frequency Interference (RFI).
- Microwave Frequency Interference (MFI).

For the purposes of this book we will use EMI to cover all of these effects. The health effects of electromagnetic interference are commonly found documented as:

- Electromagnetic Hypersensitivity (EHS).
- Electro-Hyper-Sensitivity (EHS).
- Electrical Sensitivity (ES).
- Electro-Sensitivity (ES).
- Radio Wave Sickness (RWS).
- Rapid Aging Syndrome (RAS).
- Electrical Poisoning.
- Electronic Poisoning.
- Wireless Poisoning.
- Radiation Poisoning.
- Radiation Sickness.

For the purpose of this book we will use the term Electromagnetic Hypersensitivity (EHS), as they are all essentially the same thing. The strange thing about EHS is that many people have it, but very few of them realize that it is EHS that is causing their problems. EHS has not been publicized well and even many doctors do not appear to be aware of it. Strange, considering the amount of electrical, electronic and wireless products that we are now exposed to.

EHS is somewhat of an "Inconvenient Truth" and if it became widely accepted that it was causing human health problems, then many things would have to change. Industry and governments do not like change and in order to avoid it, it is far easier to deny it. For this reason, you should be aware of your environment and of EHS so that you can stay safe until it does become widely acknowledged as being the problem that it is.

The symptoms of it can be:

133

- Neurological:
  - Headaches.
  - Dizziness.
  - Nausea.
  - Difficulty concentrating.
  - Memory loss.
  - Irritability.
  - Dementia.
  - Depression.
  - Anxiety.
  - Insomnia.
  - Fatigue.
  - Weakness.
  - Tremors.
  - Numbness.
  - Tingling.
  - Seizures.
  - Paralysis.
  - Psychosis.
  - Stroke.
- Cardiac:
  - Palpitations.
  - Arrhythmia.
  - Pain or pressure in the chest.
  - Low or high blood pressure.
  - Slow or fast heart rate.

- Respiratory:
  - Shortness of breath.
  - Sinusitis.
  - Bronchitis.
  - Pneumonia.
  - Asthma.
  - Flu-like symptoms.
  - Fever.
- Dermatological:
  - Skin rash.
  - Itching.
  - Burning.
  - Facial flushing.
- Opthalmological:
  - Pain or burning in the eyes.
  - Pressure in or behind the eyes.
  - Deteriorating vision.
  - Floaters.
  - Cataracts.
- Muscular & Skeletal:
  - Muscle spasms.
  - Altered reflexes.
  - Muscle and joint pain.
  - Leg or foot pain.
  - Arthritis.
  - Swollen joints.
  - Joint irritation.

- Others:
  - Sexual problems.
  - Digestive problems.
  - Abdominal pain.
  - Enlarged thyroid.
  - Testicular or ovarian pain.
  - Dryness of lips, tongue, mouth or eyes.
  - Great thirst.
  - Dehydration.
  - Nose bleeds.
  - Internal bleeding.
  - Altered sugar metabolism.
  - Immune abnormalities.
  - Redistribution of metals within the body.
  - Hair loss.
  - Pain in the teeth.
  - Deteriorating fillings.
  - Impaired sense of smell.
  - Ringing in the ears.

Exposure to high frequencies may cause:

- Irregular heartbeat.
- Pains.
- Allergies.
- Miscarriages.
- Birth defects.

- Childhood leukemia.
- Brain tumors.
- Reproductive tumors.
- Cancers.
- Infertility.
- Depression.
- Chronic Fatigue Syndrome (CFS).
- Fibromyalgia.
- Gulf War Syndrome.
- Alzhiemer's disease.
- Parkinson's disease.
- Lou Gehrig's disease.
- Behcet's disease.
- Sexual arousal.
- Aggression.
- Hearing things. (Loud bangs, high pitched buzzing, low frequency hum)
- Smell of smoke when there is no smoke.

Dr. Jim Burch PhD of the Cancer Prevention and Control Program at the University of South Carolina, has documented the biological effects of radio frequencies on the human mind and body as:

- **Cell proliferation (Increased ODC activity).**
- **Ion flux across biological membranes (Ca^{++}).**
- **DNA damage (Comet assay is an example).**
- **Gene expression (Oncogenes, stress proteins).**

- **Altered enzyme activity (Radical pairs).**
- **Immune system perturbations.**
- **Endocrine disruption (Melatonin for example).**
- **Altered blood-brain barrier.**
- **Autonomic nerve function (EEG, ECG).**
- **Sleep or circadian rhythm disruption.**
- **Headaches, neurological effects.**
- **Reproduction disorders.**
- **Carcinogenesis (Brain, leukemia).**

EMI can be classed as narrow-band or wide-band:

Narrow-band EMI sources can be:

- Smart meters/smart devices/automatic meter readers (AMR)/advanced metering infrastructure (AMI) utility wireless networks.
- Two way radios (transceivers).
- Cordless phones, mobile phones and cell phones.
- Wireless scanners and wireless checkout devices.
- Radio frequency identification devices (RFID).
- Wi-Fi networking.
- Television and radio transmission towers.
- Cell phone towers.
- RADAR systems.
- Rural internet and satellite internet.

Here are some sources of wide-band EMI:

- Computers.
- Cathode ray tube (CRT) TV's.
- Digital flat screen TV's.
- Power lines.
- Electric switches and relays.
- Electric motors.
- Variable frequency drives.
- Thermostats.
- Bug zappers.
- Inverter systems.
- Florescent lights.
- Compact florescent lights (CFL).
- Light emitting diode (LED) lights.
- Neon signs.
- Stereo systems.
- MP3 players.
- Electronic lamp dimmer switches.
- Cars.
- Transportation systems.
- Electric and electronic toys.
- Battery powered watches.

Most digital equipment will have broadband emissions from it. If it is switching a large amount of power, then it may produce large amounts of electromagnetic interference.

There was a shift that occurred largely in the 1980's from analogue electronics to digital electronics. Analogue

electronics did not have a digital microprocessor chip in it and was made out of many basic electrical and electronic components. More importantly, it did not have the high speed pulsing that characterizes digital electronics. It is this high speed pulsing that causes digital electronics to be generally very high electromagnetic interference producing equipment.

The pictures on the following pages show the effects of electromagnetic interference on the human body voltage.

The Human Body Voltage

The human body voltage appears like a capacitor charging and discharging when in contact with conductive flooring that is electrically grounded with stray voltage.

The Human Body Frequency Spectrum

A Fast Fourier Transform (FFT) reveals the many frequencies
contained within the human body. Zero Hertz is at the bottom
and the high frequencies are at the top.

Digital electronics uses electrical square waves to drive it. A square wave is one of the dirtiest electrical waves and as such it has many harmonics associated with it. Harmonics are the many different frequencies of sine waves that must be added together to produce the square wave. Basically, if you have a 60 Hertz square wave, then it will contain many higher frequencies of sine waves to produce it. They may be thousands of times higher in frequency than the wave that they are part of. It is for this reason that a standard AM radio when tuned into static can detect electrical noise. It is the harmonics that it is detecting in the square wave.

Computers function on high speed switching of square waves. For this reason you will find some very interesting microwave, radio, electric and magnetic fields around them. The fields vary with the age of the computer and the different brands of computers. Laptop computers can be a particular problem due to the electronics being located below the keyboard and mouse pad. Some of these areas underneath can have very high levels of EMI producing electronics! It is best with a laptop computer to switch to a large font on the display, push the laptop back and use a separate keyboard and mouse to control it. You should avoid putting it on your lap.

Compact florescent lights appear to produce radio waves from their power switching electronics. These radio emissions appear to vary between the different sizes of bulbs and also how old they are. It is not a good idea to bring radio frequency producing equipment into your environment and for this reason I advise people against using these products. Testing has shown that these products can couple their electromagnetic fields into water and cause stray voltage effects. This is a concern due to the human body being between 70% to 90% water, depending on age. Light emitting diode (LED) bulbs appear to exhibit similar effects.

Florescent tanning booths and beds may be an electromagnetic interference hot zone and should probably be avoided. The tanning light spectrum may be an issue as well.

Toxic Health © Steven Magee

Some of the new digital televisions (TV) appear to be producing levels of electromagnetic interference that are affecting peoples health. I measured electromagnetic interference that was produced by my digital TV at a distance of fifty feet away from it! The electromagnetic interference that this particular 32" LCD flat screen TV was producing appeared to be of an interference type of radiation. There were pockets of low and high interference AM radio frequencies throughout the home. I had noticed plant deformity and leaf tip problems in the plants in the room of the digital TV which may be linked to the electromagnetic interference. The interesting thing about discontinuing the use of my digital TV was that plants started to grow in my garden that had appeared dormant for years! Plasma TV's appear to be the worst offenders of the new digital TV's with large electromagnetic interference fields around some of them.

It has been noticed that intensive care patients are leaving the hospital with brain problems that were not there prior to their treatment. It is likely to be an effect of electromagnetic interference exposure. Around an intensive care bed you will typically find many electronic displays that are all emitting EMI. Many hospitals now use wireless networking and there may be numerous wireless devices all transmitting very close to the patients brain. Long term exposure to EMI is known to do strange things to the brain including brain fog, headaches, fuzzy thinking, and memory loss. Indeed, the most wireless devices that I have ever seen in one place was in the maternity ward of Tucson Medical Center! The worst example of a really poor wireless device location was placing a wireless network router directly over the new born baby's cot!!!

Solar photovoltaic (PV) power systems on the roofs of residential homes may be an issue. The inverter system that converts the direct current electricity from them into alternating current appears to cause electromagnetic fields to occur on the equipment. The large scale adoption of solar photovoltaic systems in the home has not yet been around long enough to fully understand the health risks that they may present.

Due to the advent of digital equipment, the electrical circuits of the home may need to have line terminators installed in them. Line terminators prevent digital reflections from occurring on the home wiring. Essentially, it is an electrical noise reduction technique that can be used to help prevent the home wiring from emitting radio waves.

The radial electrical circuit is shown on the next page. The last socket may now need a line terminator installing into it to terminate the circuit to prevent electronic noise reflections from occurring. A line terminator is generally a small capacitor in parallel with a high impedance bleed resistor. This would be connected across the live and neutral terminals of the final socket in the radial circuit.

Terminating Radial Circuits

Radial electrical circuits may need line terminators installing at the last outlet.

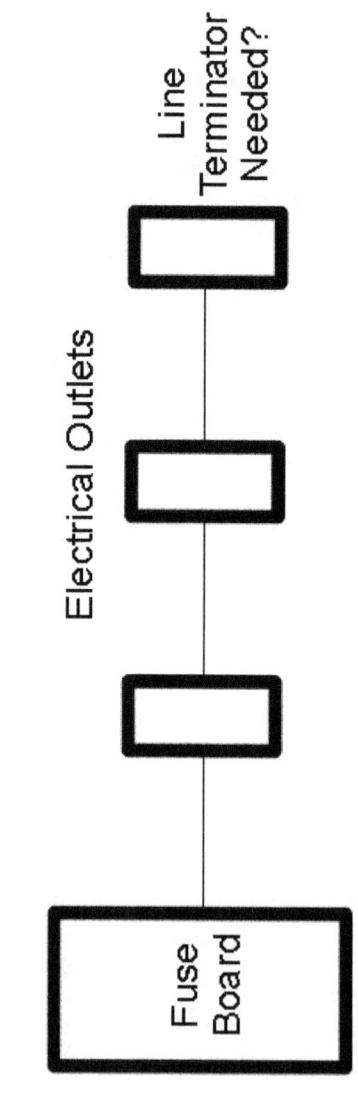

Line terminators prevent frequency reflections from occurring on the circuit. A line terminator is generally a capacitor and a resistor.

Cars and transportation systems can have high amounts of EMI associated with them. In the past this came from their ignition systems and could be heard on the car radio as a buzzing sound that would increase in line with the revolutions per minute (RPM) of the car engine. Today, there is likely to be more electromagnetic interference from the electronic systems of the car and this may include:

- Radio frequency identification devices (RFID).

- Hybrid drive system.

- Electric drive system.

- Engine computer system.

- Global Positioning Systems (GPS).

- Alternating current inverter system.

- Entertainment systems.

- Cell phone charger.

- Cell phone.

Using your cell phone in the car is a bad idea due to the radiation reflections that may occur. This may raise the radiation environment in the car and may cause interference effects that may be harmful to human health. Not to mention the distraction effect that may lead to a collision!

Electromagnetic interference is occurring with motorbikes and appears to be much stronger due to the compactness of a motorbike. Many motorbikes have their electronic systems and battery mounted under the seat and this area may emit the most electromagnetic interference into the rider. More details on this can be found in the book "Motorcycle Cancer?" by Randall Dale Chipkar.

The move to hybrid and electric cars appears to be taking place with little concern to the electromagnetic interference environment inside the car. There are reports of people detecting electromagnetic interference fields within these cars that can far exceed the 2 milli-gauss magnetic fields that the International Agency for Research on Cancer (IARC) have set as their limit for constant magnetic field level for safe human health. Other people have noticed that their children appear fatigued on a long drive in a hybrid car as opposed to a normal car. Hybrids and electric cars appear to emit high electromagnetic interference during acceleration that may be around 100 milli-gauss and up to 30 milli-gauss when cruising. Constant fields of 2 milli-gauss and above should be avoided due to the elevated cancer risk.

It is well known that frequent travelers have a high obesity risk. Transportation systems of all types can produce high electromagnetic interference environments. Planes, buses, streetcars and trains may be filled with electromagnetic interference and it is added to by people using their electronic devices on them.

Electronic lamp dimmers are one of the biggest culprits for producing electromagnetic interference effects within the home. I was quite surprised to find that a large and extensive electromagnetic field that I was detecting throughout a home was coming from a lamp dimmer! You should avoid these products and use the three way filament light bulbs instead.

Microwave ovens can produce similar effects. I have detected radio, microwave, electric and magnetic fields around these and, as such, I no longer use one. They make cell phones look safe!

People have started to realize that computer Wi-Fi networks, cell phone networks, DECT cordless phones, and the like are all causing biological problems.

When reviewing the Popular Science article "*The Man Who Was Allergic to Radio Waves*" we find that Per Segerback "*noticed his first symptoms -- dizziness, nausea, headaches, burning sensations and red blotches on his skin -- in the late 1980s, a decade into his telecommunications research work. All but two of the 20 or so other members of his group reported similar symptoms, he says, although his were by far the most severe. His EHS worsened and now, he says, even radar from low-flying aircraft can set it off."*

Electromagnetic Hypersensitivity (EHS) has been extensively documented in plants and trees around these electromagnetic fields. The biological effect in plants and trees is not new, it was extensively researched and documented by Dr. John Nash Ott in the 1950's. Indeed, I have grown plants in electromagnetic fields that exhibited the growth defects that he documented.

This is shown on the next page. The three plants all looked the same when I bought them. They are all Dieffenbachia's (Dumb Cane) and they all looked like the bushy one on the left. The center plant changed its growth in a Wi-Fi and AC voltage field location. The right plant changed its growth in a radio wave field that was produced by a 32" LCD digital television and now has very small and glossy green leaves with no patterning, as shown in the following picture. As you can see, they look like completely different species of plants and I call them my "Frankenstein" plants!

Electromagnetic Interference Effects in Plants

Exposure to EMI can cause plant deformity and growth defects. The leafy Dieffenbachia plant on the left is how the spindly ones to the right used to look before EMI exposure.

Dieffenbachia Leaves

On the left is a normal fully grown Dieffenbachia leaf. On the right is a fully grown Dieffenbachia leaf from the plant in the EMI field produced by my 32" LCD TV.

The switched mode power supply (SMPS) has replaced the traditional heavy block transformer that products used to be supplied with. This is a concern, as the switched mode power supply creates far more dirty electricity effects than the traditional transformer power supply. Indeed, some switched mode power supplies can completely fill the home with electromagnetic interference! Switched mode power supplies are poorly tested, inadequately regulated and are unfortunately powering most of the electronic products that you are purchasing that you plug into electrical sockets. It is likely that they will become highly regulated by the government in the future and I recommend that you should avoid buying electronic products until that occurs.

Babies and children are the most sensitive to the effects of EMI and particular attention should be paid to their environments. In a home with children you should avoid:

- Ionizing smoke detectors.

- Wireless baby monitors.

- Electrical and electronic toys.

- Radio controlled and wireless toys.

- Train sets and car race tracks that may produce sparks.

- Battery operated wristwatches.

- Avoid placing the baby to sleep on a party wall with your neighbor as you will not know what EMI producing equipment is on the other side of that wall.

- Avoid placing the baby to sleep near an electrical outlet.

- Avoid having electrical cables running along the floor where the baby may crawl.

- Avoid letting a baby crawl on a floor that may have electrical cables running underneath it. (Upper story of a home).

- Avoid living in apartments, as these present the biggest electromagnetic interference risk from the neighbors around you. A detached house is far better.

- Avoid letting a baby crawl on any type of electrically conductive flooring, such as tile or concrete.

- Keep babies and children away from electrical, electronic and wireless equipment in general.

Power lines and poles running through the streets is a bad idea. They have a number of problems that may lead to illness:

- **Magnetic fields.**

- **Electric fields.**

- **Electrostatic fields.**

- **Electrostatic attraction.**

- **Radio wave emissions.**

- **Plasma emissions.**

- **Ion emissions.**

- **Nitrogen emissions.**

- **Ozone emissions.**

- **Reflection and interference of sunlight.**

- **Reflection and interference of radio and microwaves.**

- **AC electrification of the ground around them (stray voltage, stray current, stray frequency).**

The utility power lines have setbacks that apply to them and for 13,800 volt AC lines, this setback is typically thirty feet either side of them. Building of homes and offices in these setbacks is generally not allowed due to the high electromagnetic fields that are present within the setback. The larger the voltage, the larger the setbacks become. Power line set backs can be several hundred feet wide on the high voltage transmission systems.

Power line radio emissions may be erratic, occurring only at certain times of the day or during certain weather conditions. They are generally caused by the induction of electrical energy into the surrounding metalwork on the power pole that can cause sparks to jump between the metalwork. A failing or dirty insulator may have a similar effect. When a power line starts to emit radio waves, these radio waves may extend beyond the power line set back. The radio waves cannot be heard or felt and a standard AM radio tuned to static (no radio station) can generally be used to detect them. Exposure to these radio waves may lead to Electromagnetic Hypersensitivity (EHS).

While developing the power line section of this book, I spent three hours each night for two nights examining the power poles and power lines in the area of my home. I noticed the following conditions occurring over the following weeks:

- **Headaches.**

- **Insomnia.**

- **Fatigue.**

- **Sore throat.**

- **Irregular heartbeats.**

- **Intestinal pains.**

- **General poor health.**

- **Heightened sexual desire occurred in the first few days after testing was finished, it appeared to be a side effect of electromagnetic interference withdrawal.**

You should not spend time directly under power lines, as this will put you into what appears to be a plasma field. Plasma is the fourth state of matter and under the power lines is an invisible flow of energy between the lines and the ground.

The electrostatic field is what appears to light up florescent tubes that are held near to power lines. It is a strange sensation to walk into a high powered electrostatic field as it is this field that makes your hair start to react. Nikola Tesla was trying to develop wireless lighting products using this field. We are fortunate that he never achieved his dream, as he may have made many people sick with his wireless lighting system. Nikola Tesla did end up being regarded as "nutty" and exposure to the electrostatic field may have been one of the things that was affecting him.

During my research into power lines producing AM radio frequencies, I noticed the reflection effect. The cell phone tower microwave signals seem to be interacting with the power lines and may be producing pockets of AM radio frequencies that can be picked up on a standard AM radio tuned to static. If you were in one of these pockets for an extended time period, you may develop Electromagnetic Hypersensitivity.

The following pages demonstrate the various effects of power lines.

Power lines and poles can have many types of large fields around them. "Dirty electricity" effects may cause extensive radio wave fields.

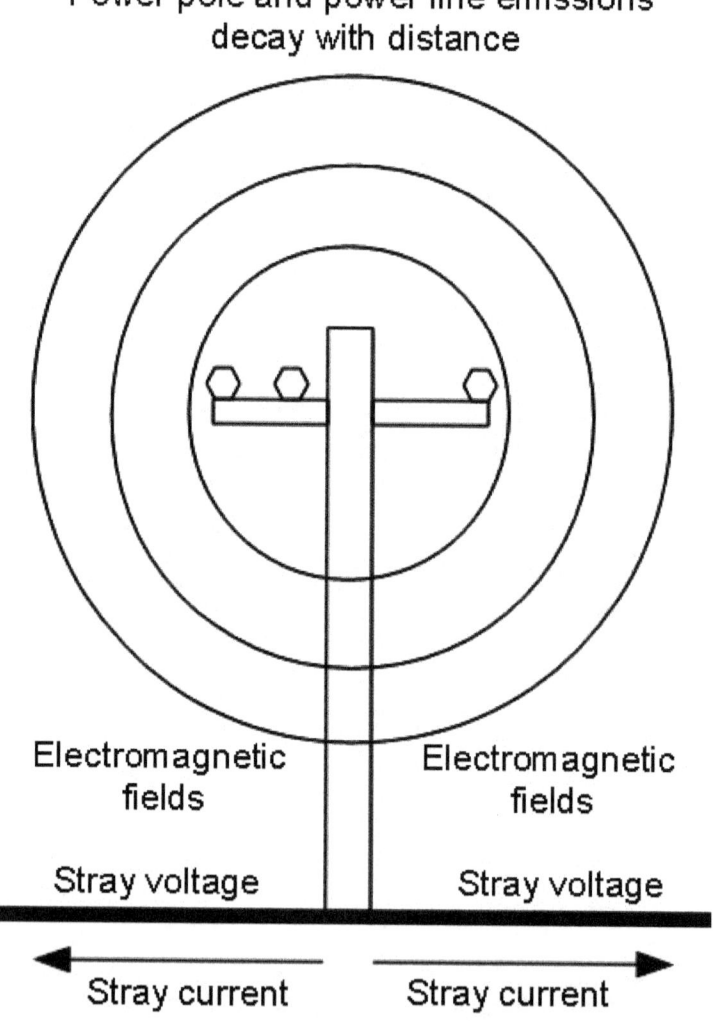

Power pole and power line emissions decay with distance

Electromagnetic fields

Electromagnetic fields

Stray voltage

Stray voltage

Stray current

Stray current

Power Pole Metal Work

Induction effects in power pole metal work may cause sparks to jump between it which will cause radio wave emissions to occur. Dirty and defective insulators do the same.

Power lines and poles can emit plasma and ions. The high voltage causes the electrostatic attraction effect. Power lines and poles have fields that extend out from the area that set backs should be applied to, to protect human health.

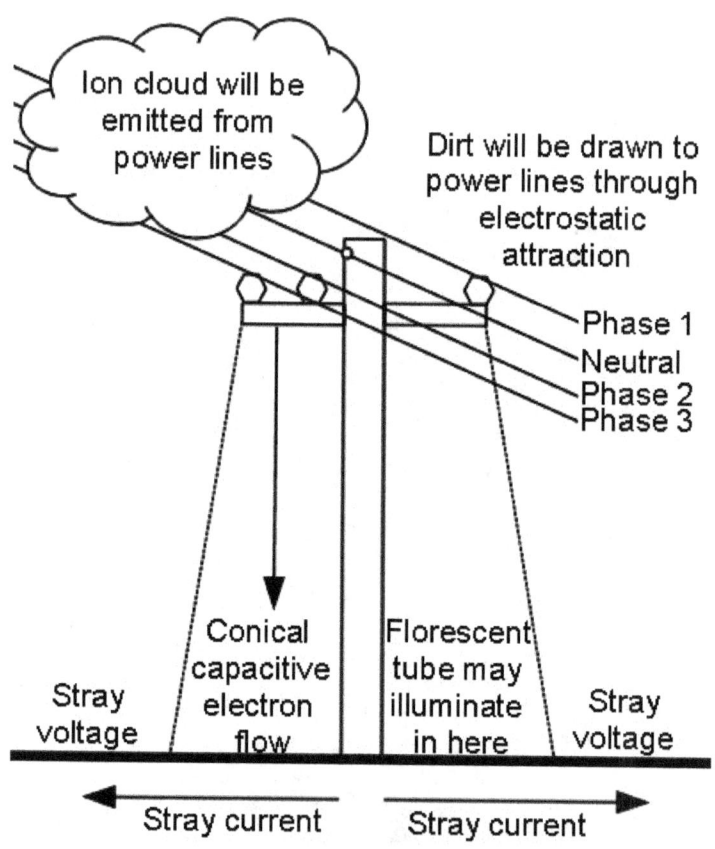

Power Line and Pole Solar Interference

The power poles and lines can interfere with the solar radiation transmission when in front of the Sun.

Toxic Health © Steven Magee

Power Line Reflections

Power lines may cause radio and microwave reflections and interference effects to occur.

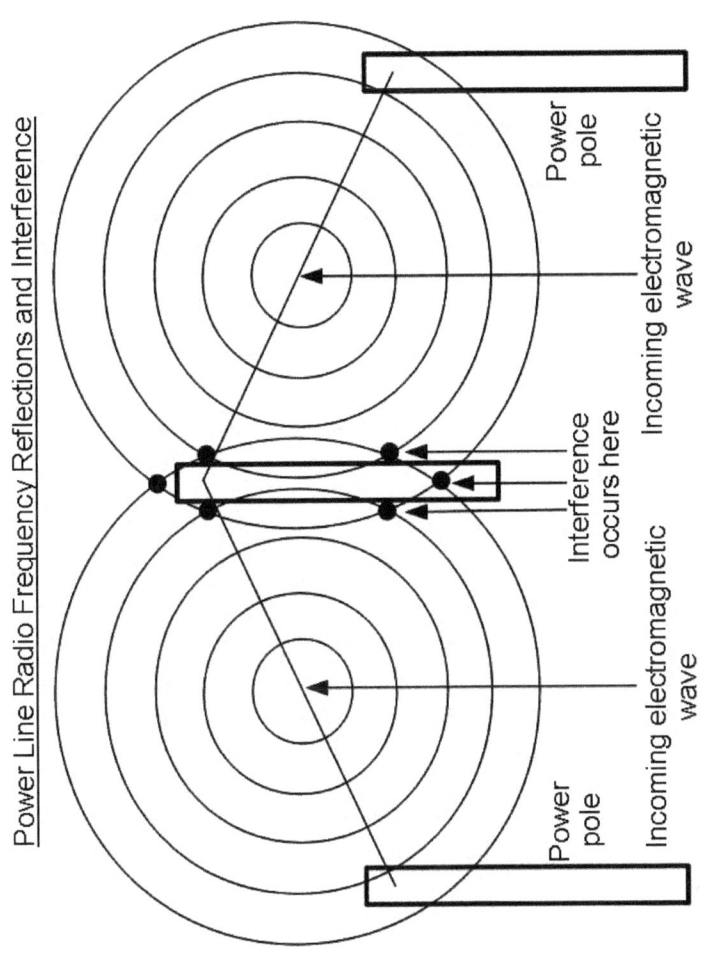

Dr. Phillip Stoddard, Professor of Biological Sciences at Florida International University, has done extensive research on utility power lines. He has found significant health risks from their presence:

- **The closer you live to a power line, the more likely you are to develop Leukemia.**

- **Living in a magnetic field of 3.5 milli-gauss doubles the Leukemia risk.**

- **Living within 0-50 meters of a power line doubles the risk of Alzhiemer's Disease and presents a 1.5 increased risk of developing Senile Dementia.**

- **Burying the power lines brings the magnetic fields closer.**

I do not recommend that you spend significant time underneath high voltage power lines, as you may be getting a free radiation treatment! They really should be fenced to keep people from venturing under them, especially young children. You should not buy a home that is underneath them if you value your health, as many people have become sick in such homes.

A common problem on buried power lines is the corrosion of the concentric neutral. The concentric neutral is the wire that you see wrapped around the outside of the utility cable that comes down the power pole. If this corrodes, then the neutral starts to become high impedance and this will cause current to increase though the ground. Basically, corrosion of the concentric neutral will electrify the surrounding ground and is clearly a human health hazard. Many people have been electrocuted by corroded neutrals after rains, due to the ground becoming more conductive to the stray electricity. Faulty insulation on the live conductor that causes leakage currents will have a similar effect.

It is not a good idea to live near to electrical equipment. The following locations should be avoided if you value your health:

- **Streetlights.**
- **Power lines.**
- **Power poles.**
- **Transformers.**
- **Substations.**
- **Switch yards.**
- **Power generation plants.**

The areas in the vicinity of these may have large amounts of stray voltages, stray frequencies and stray currents. This is shown in the next diagram.

Stray Voltage, Stray Current and Stray Frequency

Substation,
power pole,
streetlight,
transformer,
or ground
rod

The earth around electrical equipment is commonly electrified by ground rods. You should avoid coming into contact with electrified earth, as it is a human health hazard. You should keep children away from these areas.

The electrical power system in your home may also affect your health. Around electrical fuse boards there may be very high microwave and radio fields, magnetic and electric fields, and stray voltage/current/frequencies. The electromagnetic interference is a function of:

- The quality of the utility power.
- The electrical equipment that is connected to the fuse board.
- Smart/AMR/AMI utility transmitting electrical meters.
- The type of structure that it is mounted to.
- The quality of the grounding system.
- The construction of the electrical fuse board.
- The routing of the cables that connect to the equipment.
- The presence of an alternate energy system (such as solar photovoltaics or wind turbines).

It may be possible that Leukemia in children is linked to the location of the fuse board on the home. The health of babies and children is a particular concern with the advent of Smart/AMR/AMI transmitting electrical utility meters, as they broadcast wireless radiation into their surrounding environment. Babies and children are the ones who are most affected by these effects.

Some fuse boards may need filters installing and line terminators on their radial circuits. These are important in areas that have electrical power quality issues (Dirty electricity).

The location considerations for electrical fuse boards and associated equipment is shown in the following two pictures.

Electrical Fuse Boards

These should not be mounted in human habitation areas due to the fields that extend out from them that may include wireless radio frequency transmitting fields. An ideal location is on the side of the garage.

Bad Fuse Board Location

Unfortunately, the fuse board in the previous picture was located directly behind the master bed! Electrical fuse boards should not be mounted on human habitations.

The utility supplies a combined ground (earth) and neutral connection to your home that splits into the ground (earth) and neutral connection at your fuse board. The ground rods that you may see near fuse boards are to effectively ground this combined ground (earth) and neutral cable to the ground potential of the property. The voltage on the ground (earth) and neutral connections will rise up and down in proportion to the load on the electrical system in your area if it is not grounded properly by both the utility and the homeowner.

You should remember that the electrical ground (earth) connection in your home or office connects directly to the neutral transformer winding connection that is supplying the electricity. It may be carrying an AC voltage!

This is shown in the diagram on the next page.

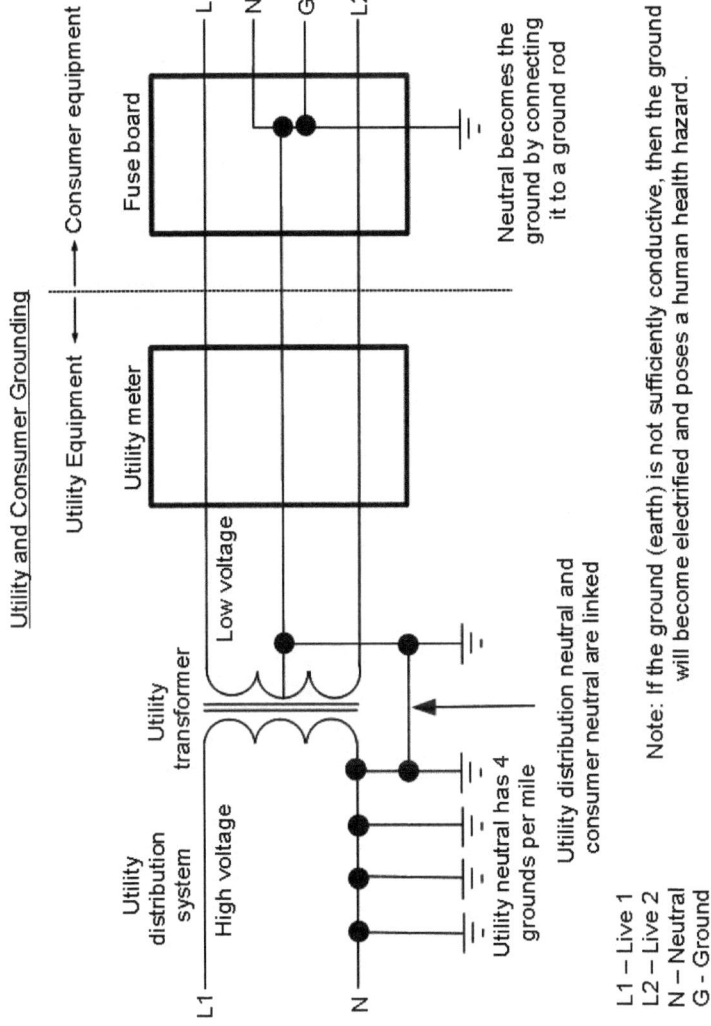

Utility and Consumer Grounding

The concept of grounding is quite interesting. The electrical system was originally designed to be a one wire supply system with an earth return through grounding rods. It was only when people started to get shocked by the electrified earth that a return wire was also installed, which we now call the neutral. However, the ground rods remained and if the neutral is higher in voltage potential than the ground, then it will feed AC voltage and current into the ground. In other words, the ground rods electrify the ground with AC electricity! This is a particular problem anywhere where the ground is a poor conductor of electricity, such as the dry desert southwest USA.

You should be aware that anywhere that a ground rod is installed, that there may be AC voltage, frequency and current in the vicinity of it. The electrification of the earth may extend several hundred feet from the ground rods. You should keep your shoes on and keep children and pets away from these areas. AC electrification of the earth commonly occurs around fuse boards, streetlights, pad mounted transformers, power poles and lines, and electrical substations too! People who walk their dogs are at particular risk from these energized earth effects.

A utility electrical substation diagram is shown on the next page. The substation relies on an earth (ground) return path for the electricity and as such, the area around electrical substations may have large amounts of stray voltage, stray currents and stray frequencies present.

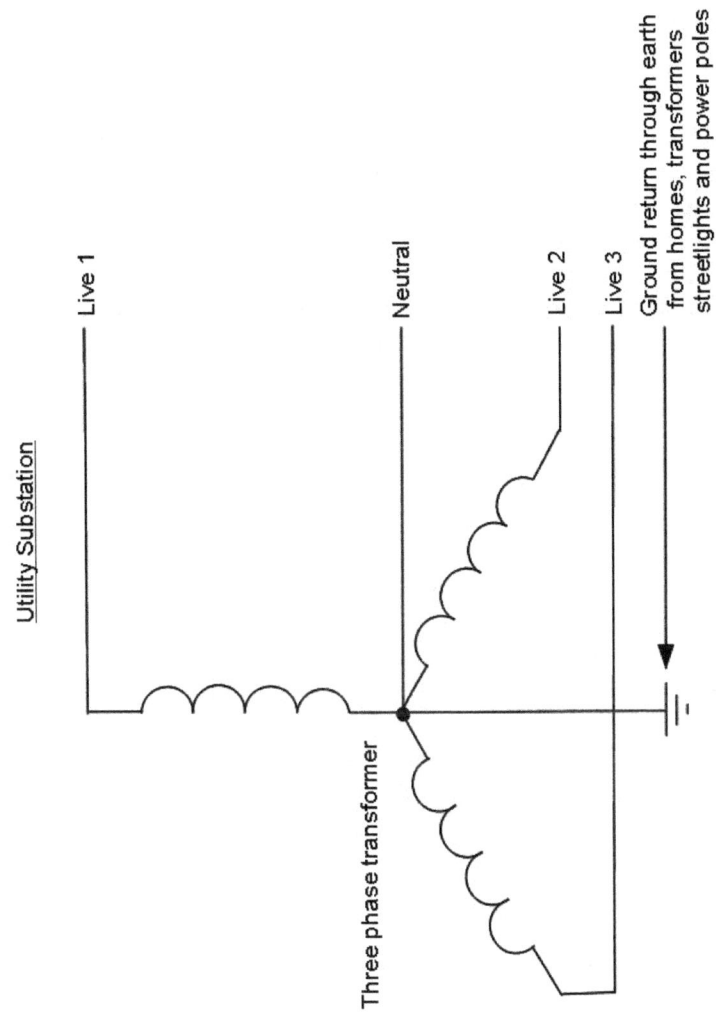

Grounding electrical systems at the home can create voltages in the home that are commonly referred to as "stray voltage". Stray voltage is a well known effect in the diary industry and it can wreak havoc on the health of farmers, their families, and their livestock. As one farmer reports "*It's a slow, painful tortuous death, is what it is for them,*" said Siewert, who with his father, Harlan, owns Siewert Holsteins in Zumbro Falls. "*It's like watching someone die of AIDS.*"

One of the things that has caused stray voltage to become prevalent in the human environment is the widespread adoption of plastic services to homes. In the past, the plumbing was cast iron drains, galvanized steel supply pipes and copper tubing. All of these were relatively good conductors of electricity and supplied good grounding to the home. This has changed and plumbing is now commonly plastic, which is an insulator to electricity. Unfortunately, you may still find that the water in the plastic drains is electrified from the sewer in the street which in turn will electrify your toilets, showers, basins and baths. It is not a good idea to be urinating into an electrified toilet!

The stray voltage effects are shown on the following pages. The next picture shows the Amprobe 5XP-A multimeter logging the maximum voltage. The following diagram shows the stray voltage in my garden as measured in the evening at my home during September 2011 in Arizona, USA. As you can see, there is an AC voltage gradient from the ground rods at the front of the home to the back of the home where the reference ground rod is installed. The 8 foot long reference ground rod is installed well away from the home and electrical systems. There are no electrical connections to it.

Measuring Stray Voltage

The Amprobe 5XP-A multimeter is logging voltage values of the electrical outlet ground pin (Right probe) to the garden ground at the back of the home (Left probe).

Garden Stray Voltage

• 8 foot reference ground rod

0.028V •

• 0.079V

Live = 124 volt
Exterior Neutral = 1.000 volt
socket Ground = 1.000 volt

0.109V •

• 0.183V

0.411V •

• 0.448V

Home

0.411V •

• 0.495V

Fuse board and
ground rods

Stray voltage measurements in the garden using an
Amprobe 5XP-A multimeter. As can be seen, there is a
voltage gradient through the property.

174

During logging both current and voltage with an Amprobe 5XP-A multimeter in August and September 2011, these are the range of values that I recorded at my home:

- 0.07 to 1.66 volts.

- 2.7 to 55 milli-amps.

- 60 Hertz AC.

- Low values occurred near sunrise, high values occurred between 16:00 to 20:00 mid-week.

- The electrical distribution network had high loads due to air conditioning loads running in the summer heat.

It is interesting to note that for electrocution to occur in water, the following conditions must exist:

- Assuming a wet human body resistance of 300 ohms.

- Muscle control in the human is lost at between 6 to 30 milli-amps.

- 1.8 to 9 volts of 60 Hertz AC is needed.

As we can see, the conditions at my home are very close to those required for a water electrocution. If a surge from an electrical fault or lightning strike on the utility system occurred, then the conditions for a water electrocution may occur. I would be very concerned if I owned a swimming pool!

Plastic plumbing may well be hazardous to human health, as it does not ground the water contained within the pipes. As such, any plastic plumbing that is routed with electrical cables may start to couple into the electrical field of the cables. The result is the water may become electrified. You may well end up with stray voltage at your faucets, basins, showers and bathtubs! Clearly an undesirable effect. The structuring of the water that may occur has unknown health effects.

Stray voltage in the past was commonly associated with swimming pools and hot tubs, but is now rapidly becoming prevalent in many other areas throughout modern society. Have you ever wondered why competent swimmers drown in their own swimming pools? It may well be stray current that killed them, particularly if an electrical fault or lightning strike occurred in the area. Electricity easily couples into water systems and electrifies the water.

Antistatic devices (ASD) are commonly used in many industries and may present a health hazard to those who work with these. If they are connected into a poor quality grounding system, then they may well cause an AC voltage to appear on the human body. My research into this area is indicating that direct, long term exposure to a low level AC voltage may cause the human body to slowly fall into illness and perhaps onto disease. It matches the findings of the diary industry that just 0.5 volt of AC electricity exposure can lead to illness in biological systems. The effects that I noticed during two weeks of wearing an antistatic wrist strap that was connected to the electrical grounding system were:

- **Headaches.**
- **Insomnia.**
- **Fatigue.**
- **Irregular heartbeats.**

It was easily cured by removing the antistatic wrist strap. The symptoms cleared up within a few weeks. When I investigated the grounding system I found 1.5 volts of AC electricity on it when compared to the garden non-electrified ground rod and a wide range of frequencies extending into the megahertz range!

Antistatic equipment is common in the hospital operating room. Dr. William Rae determined that his allergic and neurological symptoms were caused by the electromagnetic fields in the operating room. He subsequently discovered that he was not alone in his hypersensitivity, and that there was a growing population of patients with the same condition. These people are typically told by their physicians that their symptoms are "all in their minds" and that they should seek psychiatric care.

Whether you use an antistatic device or not, you may find yourself connected into the AC supply through your environment. Walking around in your bare feet or socks on conductive flooring, such as tile or outdoors, may expose you to an AC voltage. Believe it or not, walking the dog may expose you to AC voltage through the dog lead if it is conductive! Also using any device that has a metal case and is electrically grounded through the cable may expose you to an AC voltage. Metal sewing machines, metal mobile homes, metal appliances, metal electric power tools and metal kitchen equipment can be examples of this. Anything that is conductive and electrically grounded that humans come into contact with is a potential health risk. Keeping your shoes on can reduce the risk, as can wearing electrically insulated gloves.

Plants can be affected by stray voltage and they may show retarded or accelerated growth, deformed growth or go dormant. In extreme cases they may die.

Stray voltage varies with the time of the day and can change quickly. Early in the morning it can be very low and during the peak electrical load periods, it can be very high. A multimeter with a minimum and maximum logging feature is ideal to find the range of values of stray voltage. I have found the Amprobe 5XP-A multimeter to be ideal for this purpose, as it has a 16 day battery life when using a 9 volt alkaline battery.

Whether you like it or not, stray voltage, stray currents and stray frequencies are present within your own body. The body will couple into electrical fields and this can be detected with a digital multimeter or an oscilloscope. The alternating current (AC) voltage on the human body can get

quite high, often exceeding fifteen volts when next to an AC cable. Just 0.5 volt of stray AC voltage is known to affect animals and just 2 volts of AC voltage is known to kill them! The farming industry has set an upper limit on stray voltage of 0.5 volt due to the effects that have been observed in the animals.

The electrical grounding system on my home in August and September 2011 regularly exceeded this value by three times the allowable animal contact value! I have noticed sore knees and aching bones occurring every year at summertime in my current home which I now have linked to this stray voltage effect.

To establish the biological toxicity of my electrified conductive tiled flooring, I placed three Dieffenbachia plants with their soil and roots in contact with the flooring. These were placed in the master bathroom (least electrified), front hallway, and in the kitchen (most electrified). The master bathroom Dieffenbachia grew very well, far better growth than my control plants that are grown in the extensive radio frequency fields that are present throughout my home from transmitting utility meters and distant cell phone towers. This matches what many people who use the earthing health technique report. The growth pattern degraded closer to the street that I have established is electrified with stray voltage. The worst growth was the kitchen floor plant that was very close to the utility equipment and their transmitting utility meters. There are no doubts that electrified flooring is biologically harmful and you should avoid walking barefoot or sitting on such flooring.

The following picture shows the three plants used in the electrified flooring experiment.

Electrified Flooring Experiment

From left to right we can see the degrading growth patterns of the Dieffenbachia when the roots and soil are connected to electrified flooring. The left one with the best growth patterns was connected to the least electrified floor and the right plant with the most deformed and retarded growth was connected to the most electrified floor nearest to the utility equipment.

The characteristics that are observed in animals that have been exposed to stray voltage are:

- Reduced feed and water intakes.
- Increased defecation in the milking parlor.
- Increased incidences of mastitis.
- Elevated somatic cell counts (white blood cells in the milk).
- Increased still births.
- Calves born crippled.
- Calves born blind.
- Sickly newborn calves.
- Calves dying within several days of birth.
- Crippled cows.
- Joint problems.
- Behavioral changes.
- Anxiety.
- Nervousness.
- Fatigue.
- Depression.
- Poor hair coats.
- Poor reproductive performance.
- Increased aborted pregnancies.
- Reduction in milk output.
- Depressed immune systems.
- Increased death rates.

In the human, the effects appear to be very similar:

- Changed personality.

- Degrading mental health.

- Forgetfulness.

- Anger.

- Irritability.

- Anxiety.

- Fatigue.

- Eye problems.

- Nerve tingling.

- Itchy skin.

- Joint problems, especially the hips, knees and ankles.

- Arthritis symptoms.

- Aching bones.

- Sexual problems.

- Suicide.

- The problems may appear to be seasonal or related to the time of day.

- Cancer, Fibromyalgia, Multiple Scleroses and Chronic Fatigue Syndrome are suspected to be linked to it.

The emissions from AC electricity is added to by the extensive wireless communications in use in the city environment. You will see dense concentrations of wireless transmitters in the downtown areas. Further afield, you will see transmitters on government and commercial buildings. Cell phone towers litter the landscape every few miles. High powered weather and airport radar systems are present in every major city.

Toxic Health © Steven Magee

People commonly have many wireless devices in the form of cell phones, wireless networks, cordless phones, outdoor weather stations, radio controlled toys, and so on. Many people do not even realize that the utilities have installed wireless devices at their properties in the form of Smart/AMR/AMI utility meters. "Smart Meter Sickness" is now a medical diagnosis, although not formally recognized at the time of writing! Many homes today are the equivalent of antenna parks. Indeed, many electromagnetic radiation researchers call WiFi "the cell phone tower within your home". You can find higher radiation levels near these units than you can find near cell phone towers!

Male impotence is on the rise and so are the sales of impotence curing drugs. The impotence effect was noted to occur in RADAR workers during its development. Cell phones use RADAR frequencies, as does WiFi, and most domestic wireless products. It is likely that these wireless energies are contributing to the emasculation of the modern man.

Wireless radiation is readily absorbed by the human. The human is 70% to 90% water and the microwaves that are in the environment react with water. In the communications industry, this is called "Rain Fade". When it rains, the wireless radiation power levels reduce as the rain drops absorb the energy. The human body does the same thing!

When queried about how wireless radiation affects the human mind and body, the wireless radiation industry will commonly incorrectly state that the "skin effect" protects the human. The skin effect is an observation that high frequency currents will travel down the outside of a conductor and not the center of it. This effect was noticed during the development of high frequency electricity. Melanoma is linked to the high frequency skin effect.

The human body is not a conductor, but rather a semiconductor. Different electrical process are taking place and it is clear today that the human mind and body can be greatly affected by these high frequency man-made exposures. The human skin evolved in a natural

182

electromagnetic radiation environment and is now in a very unnatural man-made one that is making many people sick.

These harmful effects can be shown by growing plants in the electromagnetic fields. Dr. John Nash Ott extensively pioneered the field of electromagnetic radiation plant growth defects and his books on the subject are an interesting read. Like Dr. John Nash Ott, I have been able to deform plants with electromagnetic fields. This is what I have established:

- Found that Smart/AMR/AMI utility transmitting meters can have a toxic effect on the various biological systems that are near to them. The harmful biological effects can occur for at least 76 feet from some of the devices and can kill plants.

- Found that the radiation emissions from certain ionizing smoke detectors can retard cellular growth and may actually kill certain types of plants.

- Found that wireless radiation puts plants into a dormant state where they follow the changes in the seasons but do not actually grow or bear fruits. They become sterile and stunted. Removing the wireless radiation exposures resurrects them.

- Found that wireless radiation affects the growth and branching structure of some plants. Plants that grow tall may instead grow low to the ground.

- Some vines will not grow into areas of biologically unnatural radiation.

- Found that wireless radiation fields are patchy and unpredictable. Just moving a few inches can be the difference between a plant being healthy or it being stunted and deformed.

- Found that pulsed radiation from wireless weather station sensors and wireless utility meters can really retard and deform plants that are close to them. In some cases they will kill the plants.

- Discovered that certain electromagnetic exposures deform and retard plant growth and when removed, the plant drops all of the previous deformed leaf growth and starts growing normal growth from the tips of electromagnetic exposed part of the plant. The previously exposed part of the plant stays bald.

- Discovered that certain plants in unnatural radiation fields will only grow leaves on their branch tips at the edge of the plant. The interior of the branches of the plant stay bald. This growth pattern rectifies itself when the unnatural radiation field is removed.

- Found that the pomegranate tree will drop all of its leaf growth when the harmful wireless radiation field is removed and put up new growth from its base. The existing branches stay bald. The following year, it will put new leaf growth on both the old and new branches and bear fruit.

- Found that certain plants in biologically unnatural electromagnetic fields will turn their normally patterned leaves into dark green glossy leaves with no patterning.

It appears that when analyzing wireless radiation exposures you should think of them as you would think of a Tesla coil. The Tesla coil was where wireless radiation devices were developed from. A Tesla coil can emit biologically harmful visible sparks over long distances, often exceeding 100 feet. Some electrical, electronic, and wireless devices appear to emit similar biologically harmful "invisible sparks" a comparable distance. I call this:

"The Tesla Coil Model of Biologically Harmful Invisible Electromagnetic Radiation"

The human mind and body cannot sense these biologically harmful invisible sparks and it slowly gets sick from exposure to them. The longer you are exposed to it, the more toxic you become. The range of these toxic electromagnetic fields varies with each device and is very unpredictable.

The leaf defects that the Dieffenbachia (Dumb Cane) plant displays in unnatural electromagnetic fields are shown in the following picture.

Leaf Deformities

The fully grown leaf deformities are shown. As you can see, a wide range of different size leaves can be generated, depending on the field type and strength that the Dieffenbachia (Dumb Cane) plant is exposed to.

Regarding wireless transmitting devices, I have found after many plant growth experiments:

- **Near exposures to transmitters are the most harmful. The most harmful transmitters that I have found are the lowest power ones that are sold to consumers as harmless wireless products! Devices that continually broadcast pulses of radiation every several seconds are the worst, such as wireless weather station sensors.**

- **Intermediate exposures are those from your neighbors wireless devices and those from Smart/AMR/AMI utility meters. These are the next worst exposures and you should be familiar with the wireless products that your neighbors have at their properties. You should consider installing electromagnetic shielding between the homes if they have harmful wireless products in use.**

- **Far exposures are those that are coming from high powered transmitters that are far away from your property. Examples of these are airport, port, and weather RADAR systems, TV and radio transmitters, government transmitters, cell phone towers, and so on. You should be aware of the locations of these to both your home and workplace. Only after working through the near and intermediate exposures should you start suspecting these as sources of your problems. Distance is your friend in the world of harmful electromagnetic radiation exposures!**

My research is indicating that home wireless devices can produce a biologically toxic field close to them. The size of this harmful field varies from device to device. Some of the harmful fields from home devices can extend at least 76 feet and the field is very patchy. Some areas are really biologically toxic. Regarding the toxicity of wireless radiation exposures from common devices in the home, a clear classification is now emerging about the level of toxicity of these devices.

The most biologically harmful fields appear to be produced by pulsed radiation devices that broadcast regularly. Smart/AMR/AMI utility meters and wireless outdoor temperature sensors are good examples. "Smart" enabled devices that are designed to integrate into your utility "Smart" meter are likely to behave in a similar fashion. Some WiFi devices and smart phones also display this behavior and it may be related to the applications that they have installed on them. Automatic door opening RADAR sensors that are common in large stores may fall into this category. Security door and active animal tracking radio-frequency identification (RFID) tags are in this category.

After this, I have WiFi router exposure rated as the next most toxic device as it is broadcasting continuously in the home and workplace, make sure you do not sit near to them. You should use your computer on a wired network connection whenever possible and turn off the WiFi. Some cordless home phones may be in this category as they appear to behave like wireless networks. Wireless game controllers and radio controlled toys are in this category.

The cell phone is in the third class of toxic devices and I recommend people to avoid them. They communicate with the cell phone tower every ten minutes or so. Each time they do so, they will fill your home with wireless radiation. If you have multiple phones in the home, then your home will be filled with wireless radiation every few minutes. Some types of cordless home phones may fall into this category.

The fourth class of wireless device appears to be devices that only broadcast a short wireless pulse when they sense an event that triggers them. A garage door open or closed sensor would fall into this category. Most wireless security sensors and wireless door chimes behave in the same way. Some wireless utility meters also can exhibit this behavior.

This is the classification that appears to be emerging for home wireless devices from most toxic to least toxic:

1. **Devices that emit regular pulses of wireless radiation at short intervals of every 60 seconds or less.**

2. **Devices that constantly emit wireless radiation.**

3. **Devices that emit pulses of wireless radiation every several minutes.**

4. **Devices that emit pulses of wireless radiation infrequently.**

If you have several wireless devices close together, then you may have to reassess which category they fall into as it will increase the frequency of wireless pulses and wireless energy power being transmitted.

The frequency that a wireless device operates on may increase the toxicity of it. The most toxic device I identified at my home was a wireless outdoor temperature and humidity sensor. It operates for about a year on two AA 1.5 volt batteries. The frequency that it operated at was 433.92 megahertz and it appeared to be deforming a wide range of plants for at least a 45 feet radius from the device.

The gas company later installed an Itron 100G gas meter that surpassed the biological toxicity of that device to the human. Installed 76 feet away from my bedroom, that device induced classic Radio Wave Sickness into me! It is listed as operating at between 908 to 924 megahertz at up to half a watt of transmission power. Half a watt is high powered for a residential application that constantly transmits pulsed radiation every several seconds. It is unfortunate that the highest powered transmitting devices at your home may actually be the utility meters that you cannot switch off!

The Itron Centron, 40G and 100G utility meters become really biologically toxic when the utility meter reading car comes through the neighborhood. It has a high

powered transmitter on it that triggers all of the Itron utility meters in the area to transmit. This is by far the most biologically toxic human radio frequency exposure that I have come across in three years of radio frequency biological research. It is orders of magnitude more toxic than anything I have experienced during my research. You should avoid being outdoors in the sidewalk on the day that your transmitting utility meters are being read by the utility company meter reading car. It is actually preferable to go into the countryside on this day to avoid the spike in radiation levels. Many people will show adverse health conditions to this exposure that may last up to a week and the long term damage is currently unknown. The utilities willfully irradiating pregnant ladies, babies and developing children in their own residential sidewalks with known biologically toxic radiation probably will go down in history as one of their greatest crimes against humanity. I would recommend that you get familiar with the following: Smart Meter Opposition Groups in the United States of America http://www.takebackyourpower.net/directory/us/

To sum up, the biological toxicity of a transmitter to a human depends on the following:

- Transmission power.
- Transmitting frequency.
- Modulation of the signal.
- Intermittent, pulsed or continuous transmission.
- Reflections and interference of the transmission.
- Distance from the base station.
- Distance from you.
- Number and types of transmitters already installed into your area.
- The number, sizes and types of metals implanted into the human body.

- Your muscle mass.

- Your physical size.

- Your age.

- Your diet.

- Your past irradiation history.

- Metal jewelery.

- For the female: metal intrauterine devices (IUD) and metal bra under wires are likely to increase the risks.

Reasonable distances to stay away from transmitting devices to reduce the known health risks that they present are:

- **High powered RADAR: 20 miles.**

- **TV or radio transmitter: 5 miles.**

- **USA large city downtown area: 5 miles.**

- **Port, airport or military base: 5 miles.**

- **Cell phone tower: 1 mile.**

- **Police or hospital transmitters: 1 mile.**

- **Transmitting utility meters: Quarter of a mile.**

- **Active RFID devices: 100 feet.**

- **WiFi router: 50 feet.**

Cell phones become more hazardous the further away from the cell tower you are, as they have an automatic transmission power control feature on them to prolong battery life. When they are near to the cell tower they transmit at low power and when they are far away, they transmit at high power. If you only have one bar displaying in your phone signal strength meter, it is likely that your phone is transmitting at the highest power level and may actually be quite hazardous to you and the people around you!

Stadiums, cinema's and densely packed cubicle offices appear to be quite hazardous due to the high power levels that many cellphones create when transmitting. The largest stadiums in the USA can hold over 100,000 people and there may be a similar number of cellphones in there. That means that a packed stadium with 100,000 cellphones has the transmission power of approximately 200,000 watts of wireless energy!!! It has been noticed that American football players are developing strange brain cancers and it may be related to this effect. Unfortunately, I have not seen any studies of similar aged regular game spectators that carry cellphones and their brain cancer types and levels. It is prudent to avoid large groupings of people in a cell phone society. The medical profession will likely call this:

Dense Population Syndrome

You should be very wary of where you keep your cellphone and men should avoid keeping it near to their testicles and women should avoid keeping it near to the breasts. You should avoid putting a cellphone in your shirt pocket or bra as it will be irradiating your breasts, heart and lungs. You most certainly do not want to sleep with your cellphone under your pillow, but unfortunately, many children do this every night. It is preferable to carry a cellphone in a separate bag away from the body. It is important to note that many cellphone manufacturers now state in their phone manuals that it must be kept away from the body by approximately half an inch for safety. This is in contrast to most people that I observe holding the phone against their heads while talking, there is no space. When in the home, use it on speakerphone and keep it far away from the bedrooms.

It is interesting to note that astronomers have always thought that a mass human radiation extinction would come from a solar flare or a supernova. Pulsars may present the biggest naturally occurring risk to human extinction, as they

behave like pulsed wireless transmitters. **As we know today, the pulsar radiation emission is far more harmful at much lower power levels than the continuous radiation emissions from the Sun or supernovas. This opens up the range of nearby astronomical objects that can threaten the Earth by orders of magnitude. As such, a human radiation extinction is far more likely to come from a pulsar than any other astronomical object!**

When we talk about extinction, we must remember that this will also affect everything on the Earth. Human survival is completely dependent on plants. Plants are affected by many forms of radiation and I have performed numerous tests that show the biologically harmful effects from man-made radiation exposures, as has Dr. John Nash Ott.

Regarding the toxicity of wireless radiation exposures, this is the official stance currently:

Lyon, France, May 31, 2011: The WHO/International Agency for Research on Cancer (IARC) has classified radio frequency electromagnetic fields as possibly carcinogenic to humans (Group 2B), based on an increased risk for glioma, a malignant type of brain cancer, associated with wireless phone use.

I have found climbing vines will not grow into areas of harmful wireless radiation and that the Golden Pothos will lose the patterning on its leaves in these fields. This is shown in the following pictures.

Golden Pothos

The Golden Pothos will lose the patterning in its leaves when in harmful wireless radiation fields. They grow dark green.

Climbing Vines

Some climbing vines will not grow into harmful wireless radiation areas. They provide an excellent indicator of the invisible patches of harmful wireless radiation that now exist.

Electrical energy interacts with the natural fields of the Earth. The human is genetically adapted to interact with natural, weak magnetic and electromagnetic fields. The cities represent the opposite of what nature created and today are an alien environment for the modern human. As such, it is reasonable to say that the modern human is an alien having developed in such an alien environment.

The alien human is revealing itself in many ways. We can see it in the dramatic rise in childhood development problems. Autism, attention deficit disorder, hyperactivity, insomnia, depression, fatigue, aggression and accelerated puberty are all problems that are prevalent in modern children. Autism is the most striking and has accelerated from being a rare problem in the 1970's where only 1 in 10,000 children were diagnosed with the condition to a common development issue where 1 in 40 boys have it today!

Autism has been following the rise in wireless communications for the last decade and this is shown in the next graph. The graph was complied from data presented by CTIA-The Wireless Association and Talk About Curing Autism (TACA). It is clearly an electromagnetic radiation disease. The longer the damaging effects of man-made electromagnetic radiation are denied, the more this graph will continue to increase. Unfortunately, the wireless radiation era is not a good time to be born into.

Copyright Steven Magee Books

Year	Autism (ratio * 20000)	Cell Phones (millions)	Cell Towers (thousands)
1998	2	44	30
2001	133.4	128	128
2006	181.8	233	196
2011	333.2	332	283

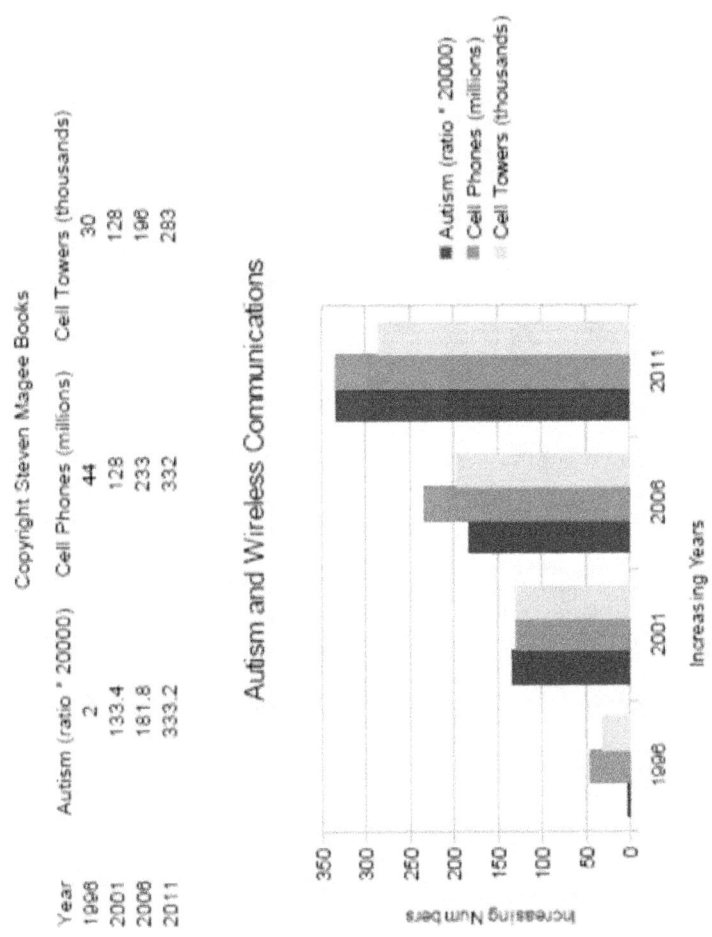

Autism and Wireless Communications

The BioInititaive 2012 report states:

The premise of this review is that although scant attention has been paid to possible links between electromagnetic fields and radiofrequency exposures (EMF/RFR) and Autism Spectrum Disorders (ASDs), such links probably exist. The rationale for this premise is that the physiological impacts of EMF/RFR and a host of increasingly well-documented pathophysiological phenomena in ASDs have remarkable similarities.

Loops are present throughout the human body and some are obvious and others are more discrete. Some of the places that you will find loops in the human body are:

- Inner Ear.
- Eye pupil.
- Eye orbit.
- Nostril.
- Spinal column.
- Collar bone.
- Circular bone surrounding marrow.
- Heart.
- Rib cage.
- Intestines.
- Kidneys.
- Ovaries and fallopian tubes.
- Hips.
- Blood cells.
- Arteries, veins, and capillaries.

Why are loops a concern? Because they may couple into the electrical fields by a process called "induction". Induction may cause electrical currents to flow within the loops when in the presence of frequency fields. Flowing currents through these loops may cause illness and disease to occur. The currents may cause localized heating, electric and magnetic fields.

Regarding the blood, the cells are known to stick together in long chains when in unnatural electromagnetic fields. The effect is known as a "rouleaux formation" and it can be undone by exposing the blood to natural sunlight.

Man-made loops may be present on the human body and we see these in various locations:

- Eye wear.
- Earrings.
- Necklace.
- Rings.
- Bangles.
- Bracelets.
- Watches.

You should also be wary of any kind of metal on the human body. In particular, the curved metal wire in under-wired bra's has already been identified to be acting as a reflector for focusing radio and microwaves into the breast tissue. Breast cancer is on the rise in young ladies who carry cellphones in their bras and the risk is increased if they have a history of chest X-rays as a teenager. Metal zippers can have similar focusing effects. The next diagram shows this effect.

A similar effect to the under-wired bra may occur in the astronomical field, but on a much larger scale. Metal observatory domes may act as reflectors that focus radio and microwaves. Any curved metal structure may exhibit this focusing effect. You should not use transmitting devices in such environments. This is shown in the following diagram.

Any metal structure may be able to cause radio and microwave reflections to occur and you should be wary of using products that create electromagnetic waves in locations such as these.

Focusing Radiation with an Under Wired Bra

Electromagnetic interference, radio and microwaves

High radiation zone

High radiation zone

Metal Dome Radiation Reflections

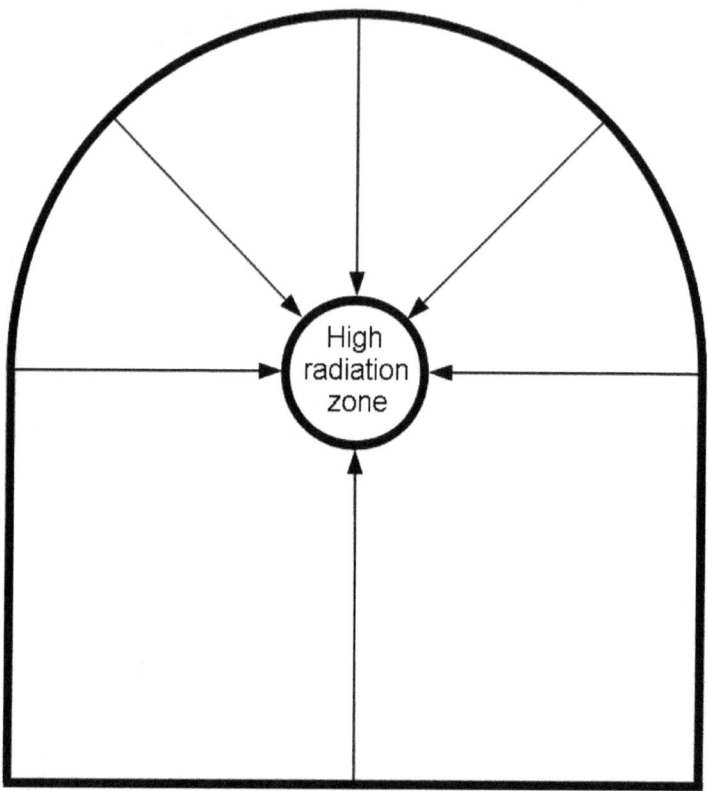

Any transmitting device in the center of the dome will create a high radiation area from the reflected waves

The human nervous system never connects in a loop and this is probably to prevent electrical induction effects from occurring in it. Instead the nerves are balanced between the left and right side of the human body, feeding out radially from the spinal cord to the various bodily systems that they connect to.

High powered alternating current electricity does not occur in nature and it is wise to exercise caution around it. There must be a reason why nature does not use it and it would be foolish to ignore this. All high powered electricity in nature is direct current (DC). The electric eel is a good example of this and it can generate a voltage of approximately 500 volts to stun its prey. Thunderstorms also produce large DC voltages of millions of volts and we see this as lightning. It appears that Edison was right to promote the use of DC electricity in the famous "War of the Currents" that he had with Tesla's AC system.

Radio waves do occur in nature and these generally are seasonal with the arrival of lighting storms. It appears that the radio waves that nature produces are a stimulant to the human mind and body for fertility and also sexual desire. Given that humans have now filled their environments with radio waves all year round, it should come as no surprise that we have seen unprecedented growth in human population over the last century. The human body may now be extremely fertile all year, as opposed to the fertility and mating cycles following the seasons in the past.

Fortunately, the human mind and body does appear to have an electrical noise reduction system built into its nervous system. The nervous system is widely acknowledged to be driven by electrical impulses, so this is not a surprise. The left part of the brain controls the right side of the body and the right part of the brain controls the left side of the body. This twist that occurs appears to be an electrical noise reduction technique that enables the body to function in high EMI environments. This is shown in the next diagram.

Human Body Electromagnetic Field Cancellation

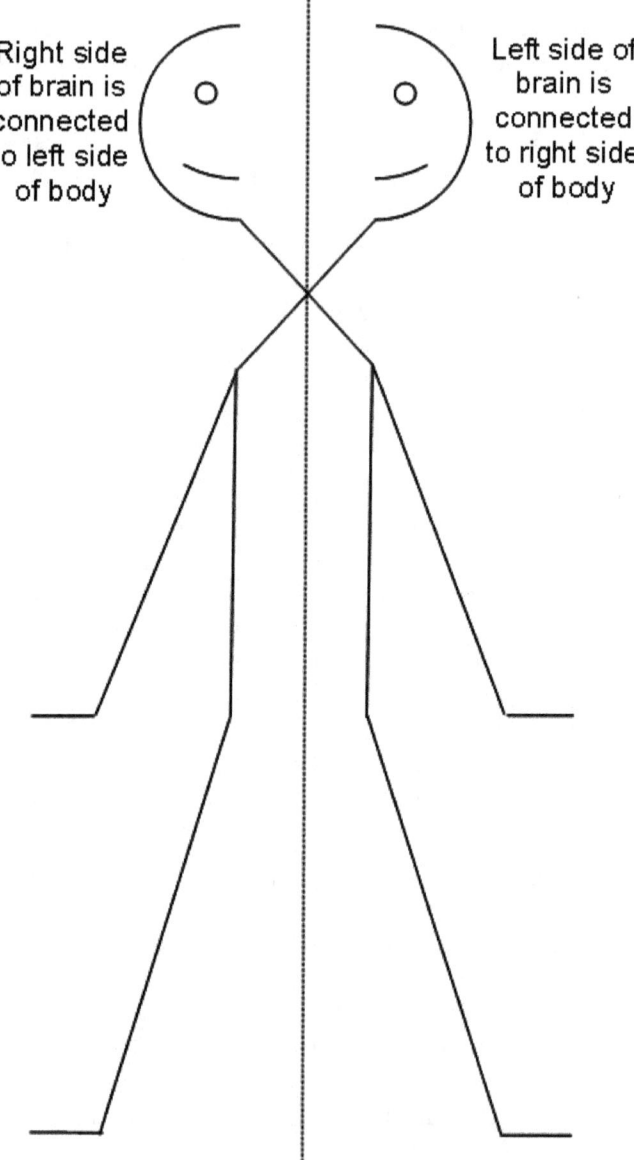

Right side of brain is connected to left side of body

Left side of brain is connected to right side of body

The nervous system uses electrical noise reduction techniques

The back and forth structures of the brain and intestines may also be an electrical noise canceling technique. The arteries and veins generally run next to each other and this is another electrical noise reduction effect. The double helix spiral in DNA creates electromagnetic shielding and nullification effects. Electrical noise reduction techniques are present throughout the body.

There are certain parts of the body that may act like antennas and these may be:

- Brain.
- Body.
- Spinal cord.
- Intestines.
- Arms.
- Legs.
- Digits.
- Hair.

It is well known that when the human is placed into an unnatural electromagnetic environment that this affects the intestinal flora. The intestines are filled with digestive microbes and the growth of these can either be retarded or accelerated by the electromagnetic fields that they are in. Retardation will bring about poor digestion and acceleration will bring on excessive gas due to overgrowth inside the intestines. I experienced the gassy overgrowth effect in one of my jobs when I was sitting next to an electrical room daily.

Fertility appears to improve away from wireless technologies. Before trying to get pregnant, I recommend that people clean up their electromagnetic environments to give their children the best chance of going to the full term of 9 months and being born into an environment that is conducive to their healthy development.

Royal Raymond Rife (May 16, 1888 – August 5, 1971) was developing frequencies of energy for medical treatments. He found that certain frequencies would alleviate certain conditions. His work appeared to evolve into what we now know today as transcutaneous electrical nerve stimulation (TENS) devices that are used to heal and radio frequency therapy that produces deep heating in the body tissues and stimulates collagen tightening, repair and regeneration.

If we take a look at the history of EMI we can see that there are definite steps in the progression of it throughout society:

- 1800's-1860's: Telegraph development. Joseph Henry invents the electric doorbell.

- 1870's: Thomas Edison develops the phonograph and starts manufacturing light bulbs. Alexander Graham Bell patents the telephone. Henry dies, aged 80.

- 1880's: Edison and Nikola Tesla are developing their electrical distribution systems. Edison sets up the first electrical utility using a 110 volt direct current (DC) system in New York City. More than 150,000 USA people are using telephones.

- 1890's: Oil and gas were starting to replace coal and wood. X-rays discovered. Tesla sets up the first alternating current (AC) utility in Niagara Falls.

- 1900's: Cars and airplanes were developing with electrical ignition systems. Most homes have electric doorbells.

- 1910's: Radio is being developed. First World War. Tesla's mental health is degrading and he is having financial problems.

- 1920's: Widespread adoption of Tesla's alternating current electrical system in cities. Leukemia is appearing in the population. The mass population is being exposed to electric lights and cinema. Bell dies, aged 75.

- 1930's: Widespread adoption of radio. RADAR and jet engine is in development. Edison dies, aged 84.

- 1940's: Widespread adoption of the alternating current (AC) electrical system in farming communities. Second World War. Development of nuclear bombs and worldwide dispersal of man-made fall-out radiation. Tesla dies, aged 86.

- 1950's: Development of the transistor and nuclear power. Extensive air testing of nuclear bombs and worldwide radiation fallout. Dr. John Nash Ott is discovering many detrimental health effects of electromagnetic radiation.

- 1960's: Widespread adoption of televisions and cars. The modern computer is being developed. The Space industry is being developed. The medical profession is trying to understand organ failure. Nuclear bomb testing moved underground to prevent worldwide radiation dispersal. Dr. John Nash Ott is discovering X-ray emissions from florescent lights and televisions.

- 1970's: Widespread use of digital watches and calculators. Adoption of international jet travel. Many communications satellites are now in orbit. Smooth float glass is becoming common in buildings. Color television became popular. Dr. John Nash Ott is discovering that electrical lighting products are changing the gender of animals and plants.

- 1980's: Widespread adoption of home and business computers, video games, video recorders and portable cassette players. Typical microprocessor speed of 1Mhz. Satellite television is in homes, as are radioactive ionizing smoke detectors. Diabetes is widespread. Cell phone towers are being constructed. Dr. John Nash Ott is discovering that the new electronic products are causing health problems in humans. Florescent lighting products are inducing cancer into his laboratory rats.

- 1990's: Widespread adoption of digital electronics into the home and workplace. Typical processor speed of 10Mhz. Cordless home and business phones that use radio frequencies are becoming popular. Coated double glazed glass is becoming commonplace in homes and businesses. RADAR systems are in use in commercial applications and weather forecasting. Autism is starting to become prevalent. Construction of International Space Station (ISS) is started. Rapid construction of cell phone towers is significantly raising the radiation levels. Dr. John Nash Ott is failing in his efforts to get his findings out to the mainstream population, media organizations will not report it.

- 2000's: Internet was widely adopted and much of commerce became conducted using it. Laptop computers and cellphones became popular. Typical processor speed of 100Mhz. Ionizing smoke detectors are installed in every bedroom. Electrical outlets are now installed every ten feet in homes. Obesity epidemic underway. Bee colonies are collapsing around the world. Fraudulent invasions of countries. Dr. John Nash Ott dies after much of his work is willfully ignored by the government, corporations, media, and research institutions.

- 2010's: GPS systems, tablet computers and smart phones became popular. Almost all young children now have cellphones, computers, and electrical and electronic toys. Children's game consoles now have wireless radiation controllers. Typical processor speed of 1 Ghz. Breast cancer is affecting 1 in 8 women. Almost all types of cancer are increasing. Autism and Attention Deficit Disorder (ADD) are widespread. Atmospheric carbon dioxide is double the historical records. Construction of the International Space Station is completed and it is the largest man-made object in orbit. The Earth is ringed in thousands of man-made satellites that are regularly eclipsing the Sun. The sky is filled with chemical trails from jet aircraft that linger for hours. Cirrus clouds have become prevalent. Cell phone coverage of 99% of the USA population is achieved with many people in multiple cell phone system transmission areas. Homes and workplaces have been turned into high powered antenna parks with the installation of radiation transmitting Smart/AMR/AMI utility meters and people are getting sick from them. The next generation of weather RADAR systems are installed into USA cities. The human electromagnetic radiation environment has never existed in the history of the world. The USA is calling itself "The Greatest Nation on Earth".

So as we can see, electromagnetic interference has been constantly changing over the last two centuries to the point where we are immersed in electromagnetic interference fields that are a soup of various forms of radiation. The biggest man-made experiment on the Earth is in full swing and you are a part of it!

So how do you prevent electromagnetic interference? The main thing that you can do is reduce your exposure by switching off as much of your electrical, electronic and wireless products as possible. You should also identify how much electromagnetic interference each of your products emits. A simple AM radio tuned to static (no radio station) can detect most electromagnetic interference fields and they are strongest at the equipment and fade with distance. De-clutter your home from these products and just have the products that you really need. Naturally, your bedrooms should be free of any electromagnetic interference producing equipment. If you are going to use electromagnetic interference producing equipment, then you should be using low electromagnetic interference versions of it wherever possible. You should consider switching off the electrical circuit breakers for rooms that you do not use and also the bedrooms. It is a good idea not to be exposed to AC electrical fields while you are sleeping. Some people actually turn off their electrical fuse board when they go to bed to effect this.

Have an electrician check your electrical ground, plumbing ground, conductive flooring, water systems, drains, and garden for stray voltage and dirty electricity effects.

If you are serious about eliminating the sources of electromagnetic interference then you may want to obtain the following items of test equipment to aid with diagnosing problems (My test equipment is in brackets):

- A portable, battery powered analogue AM radio (Sharper Image Model GFSI-0100).

- A digital multimeter with a minimum and maximum feature (Amprobe 5XP-A).

- A magnetic field, electric field, and microwave field meter (TriField Model 100XE).

- A low frequency magnetic field detector (Telephone voice pickup coil connected to a battery powered amplified speaker.)

- A battery powered oscilloscope with a Fast Fourier Transform function (FFT) (Owon PDS 5022S).

- A three axis RF meter (Tenmars TM-196).

- A battery powered LASER and RADAR detector (Whistler XTR 445).

You should make yourself aware of the peak load times of the electrical systems in your area and see if they coincide with health problems occurring:

- Air conditioning loads of summertime.

- Heating loads of wintertime.

- Industrial area load peaks are 08:00 to 17:00.

- Residential area load peaks are 16:00 to 20:00.

- Solar power systems turn on shortly after sunrise and turn off shortly before sunset with peak power being midday. On a day with broken clouds, they will produce rapid energy swings on the electricity system that will modulate the current flow in the area which may produce frequency emissions on associated electrical equipment. This effect is known to make some solar photovoltaic workers mentally and physically sick and is likely to become known as "Solar Photovoltaic Syndrome".

- Wind power peaks will coincide with the rising wind speed in the area. Wind power systems typically turn on at approximately 12 miles per hour (MPH) and generally don't make much power below 20 MPH wind speeds. They should generate significant electrical power above 30 MPH. Wind Turbine Syndrome is now a documented health condition that may occur in areas that have wind turbines installed. Denmark is considered to be the home of the wind turbine and it has seen a recent spike in its breast cancer and melanoma rates that may be related to the large number of wind turbines in that country.

You should also pay attention to where you spend time and how you feel in those environments. A long drive may bring on symptoms from exposure to car electromagnetic interference and pollution. Time spent at your job may bring on symptoms from either Sick Building Syndrome or pollution that your job exposes you to. Your employer may be avoiding informing you of known hazards of your job, as they may have seen the same thing with previous employees and know that the job is hazardous to human health. You may be the latest employee getting sick out of the many people who came before you!

Toxic Health © Steven Magee

It is an unfortunate state of affairs that we find ourselves having to do the governments job of protecting ourselves from known harm. Electrical, electronic and wireless equipment should never have been allowed into the home or workplace that may cause harm to human health. It is a sign that self regulation by industries does not work and that profits have been put before human health. With the recent environmental disasters of Hurricane Katrina in 2005, the BP Deepwater Horizon gulf oil spill in 2010 and the Fukushima nuclear disaster in 2011, we can see that the modern government systems of public protection are failing.

In this "modern" society, it is clear that you are responsible for your own health. Ultimately, if you have EHS, you may have to move to the countryside to a known low electromagnetic interference area if you are unable to clean up your environment sufficiently. Trees are excellent at suppressing electromagnetic interference due to their effective grounding. They essentially are nature's version of the Faraday Cage that is used to suppress electromagnetic interference in the engineering field.

An interesting fact that bears some thought are the differences that were observed in Edison and Tesla. Edison was developing a direct current (DC) electrical system and Tesla was developing an alternating current (AC) system. Edison was regarded as a respected businessman, while Tesla was regarded as a mad scientist. It is quite possible that the mental issues that Tesla displayed had come from exposure to his work with alternating current. Direct current that Edison was working with does not transmit through the air as well. Both men lived into their 80's and Edison was experimenting with dietary intake towards the end of his life, presumably to cure his ailments. Perhaps Edison had become a victim of exposure to Tesla's alternating current system, the very system that he had lobbied against as being a danger to human health!

It is unfortunate that these electromagnetic interference effects have occurred and we may now have widespread electrical poisoning in the modern world. An electrically

212

poisoned human is not going to think normally nor function normally. When you observe the modern population you can see that there are many different personalities around, many of which do not appear to be normal and it is probably a sign of poisoning.

Humans are displaying an addiction to electrical energy that appears to be like drug addiction. It rules their lives. Humans should be weaned off electrical energy consumption in order to reduce this unnatural dependance that has been formed. Homes should have trees placed around them to help keep them cool and reduce the air conditioning loads on the electrical grid. Ideally, homes should be located under the tree canopy.

The human mind and body cannot sense most forms of radiation. It slowly gets sick from exposure to biologically harmful forms of it. Harmful radiation comes in many forms in society:

Radio frequencies have become a plague in modern society. Many conditions are linked to it including Autism and Attention Deficit Disorder. Are you being affected? Radio Wave Sickness is well categorized today and the top reported Radio Wave Sickness symptoms in order of frequency are: Fatigue, sleep disturbance, headaches, feeling of discomfort, difficulty in concentrating, depression, memory loss, visual disruptions, irritability, hearing disruptions, skin problems, cardiovascular, dizziness, loss of appetite, movement difficulties and nausea. (Source: Symptoms experienced by people in the vicinity of a cellular phone base station, Santini 2001, La Presse Medical.) Radio Wave Sickness is commonly referred to today as Electromagnetic Hypersensitivity and how high is too high for wireless radiation exposures? People with Electromagnetic Hypersensitivity commonly report the following: 6 to 3 V/m: Too high for ambient levels. 1 to 0.3 V/m: Too high for many people. 0.1 to 0.05 V/m: Many people have symptoms. 0.02 to 0.01 V/m: Most people with EHS are okay. (Source: EMFields Acousticom 2). The Tenmars TM-196 RF meter manual states *"We recommend a maximum level of 0.614 V/m for prolonged exposure"*. It is normal to find yourself sitting and walking around in fields of wireless radiation of approximately 1 V/m in the USA. Antenna systems are commonly unseen inside buildings and various products that professional testing can reveal their presence. Invisible transmitters are called "Stealth" systems in the industry.

RADAR is found in security sensors, traffic control systems and automatic doors on many shops. It can travel for quite some distance from the RADAR device. RADAR exposure is linked to cataracts, impotence and Radio Wave Sickness.

LASER is commonly found in speed control devices. The LASER beam can travel for long distances and may be pointing at your home or workplace. LASER exposure is known to affect the eyes.

Electric fields are found anywhere there are energized electrical cables. All cables emit them. The size of the electrical field can vary with the dirty electricity on the electrical system. You may get fatigued from electrical field exposure.

Magnetic fields are created by current flow through electrical cables and they are known for their ability to affect the human mind. Strange psychological issues may show up. You will find these in your home, your workplace, your car, public transportation systems and near to power lines. Ground loops are a common problem and if you have one in your home, it may be comparable to living under a power line.

Electrostatic fields are found near to power lines. This is the field that will make the hair on your body react and stand up. It is generated by high rates of change of voltage. People who live in homes that have this field in them may slowly get sick.

Ionizing radiation sources are found in smoke detectors, X-Ray machines and some industrial meters. They are to be avoided. Ionizing radiation is regarded as the most biologically harmful form of radiation and comes from nuclear reactors.

Stray voltage/current/frequencies comes from electrical grounding systems and is known for its ability to significantly affect human health. In the home it is typically seen to electrify conductive tile and concrete flooring, metal cases of appliances, drains and the water systems of the home. Just 0.5 volt of AC electricity is known for its harmful effects on biological systems. The latest research is indicating that biological issues are being seen at just 0.01 volt of AC stray voltage exposure.

Ultraviolet (UV) and Infrared (IR) exposures come in two forms and these are increased or decreased exposures. Increased exposures occur on the outside of reflective buildings and from some types of electrical lighting products. Decreased exposure comes from filtered light through windows and also from electrical lighting products. Correct selection of electrical lighting products and window types is important in preventing Sick Building Syndrome from occurring. Dr. John Nash Ott reported cells would rupture when exposed to too much UV. This famous quote summarizes his findings: "Mal-illumination is to light as malnutrition is to food."

Electromagnetic Interference (EMI) comprises of all of the above exposures. EMI is known for its harmful health effects and is poorly regulated in the USA. There are many biologically toxic products on sale that may make you sick with long term exposure to them. EMI is so good at making people sick that the modern military weaponized it decades ago and calls them "Electromagnetic Weapons" or "Silent Weapons".

One of the beneficial effects of electromagnetic radiation are the naturally occurring Schumann Resonances. People report the use of electromagnetic waves as being beneficial to health and these devices are commonly called "Schumann Resonators" that put out the natural Schumann Resonance of 7.83 Hz. I have not met anyone yet who has successfully applied Schumann Resonances to alleviate their health conditions. I investigated the application of Schumann Resonances to the human through to the eighth harmonic and did not reach any definite conclusions. However, I have grown plants inside of a Faraday cage with a radiation source and they showed beneficial growth patterns when compared to Faraday cage plants without the radiation source. This is in line with the belief that the International Space Station has a Schumann Resonator installed in it to keep the astronauts healthy.

I applied the Schumann Resonances to the human mind by using standard electrical headphones connected to an MP3 player. The soundtrack that I developed is available commercially and is called "7.83Hz Schumann Resonance to the Eighth Harmonic". It contains harmonics of the original fundamental frequency through to the eighth. Tracks with harmonics 1, 2 or 3 may not be audible, but do produce the electromagnetic wave from the coils inside the headphones.

You need to be careful with electrical headphones, as you are applying an electromagnetic wave to the human brain. You should avoid using electrical headphones and use either speakers or air tube headsets to listen to your music. Regarding speakers, make sure that you are sitting several feet away from them due to the magnetic and electromagnetic fields that come out of them.

When applying the Schumann Resonances through electrical headphones I did notice that my sleep patterns changed and I was waking up before sunrise for a few days. I also saw some strange nerve twitching in my shoulder and headaches that cleared up after several days of continued application of the soundtrack. There appeared to be no lasting effects after I stopped applying them after one month of daily application of the resonances for two hours a day. I stopped as I was not seeing any improvement in my energy levels.

To sum up this chapter, here are the suspected health hazards of electromagnetic interference:

- Direct contact with electricity system live conductors can cause electric shock, electrical burns, and possibly death.

- Corroded utility neutrals may shock and cause electrocution.

- A surge in stray voltage may cause human electrocution in swimming pools and wet areas.

- Long term exposure to stray voltage may cause human health to degrade.

- Long term exposure to electric fields may cause human health to degrade.

- Long term exposure to magnetic fields above 2 mill-gauss may cause human health to degrade.

- Long term exposure to radio or microwave fields may cause human health to degrade.

- Long term exposure to an ion field imbalance may cause human health to degrade.

- Long term exposure to power lines may cause human health to degrade.

- Long term exposure to electricity that contains harmonics and various frequencies (Dirty electricity) may cause human health to degrade.

- Nighttime exposure may be a higher risk, due to radio waves transmitting better during this time.

- Reduction or loss of atmospheric DC voltage may cause human health to degrade.

More details on this subject can be found in the following books:

The book "Toxic Electricity" presents an analysis of the toxicity of electricity, electronics and wireless radiation.

The health effects of the AC electricity system can be found in "Dirty Electricity: Electrification and the Diseases of Civilization." by Dr. Samuel Milham MD MPH. He notes that Leukemia is almost unknown in Africa where there is minimal electrification and the disease appears to be following the progress of electrification. It was unknown by the world medical profession until the 1920's when electricity started to become commonplace.

The Earth's ground is now very different and more on this subject can be found in the book "Earthing: The Most Important Health Discovery Ever?" by Clinton Ober, Stephen T. Sinatra MD, and Martin Zucker. You need to be very careful about connecting into the ground in developed environments that have electricity, as they may have energized the ground around the electrical systems. If the ground has been energized by AC electricity, then you may get very sick by being in contact with it. Earthing the human body to the electrical system and/or electrified earth and/or cables that have radio frequencies on them may be a risky activity for long term human health.

The book "Electrocution of America: Is Your Utility Out to Kill You?" by Russ Allen documents the detrimental health effects of stray voltage/current/frequencies in the ground.

Documentation regarding the rise of electromagnetic interference pollution can be found in the following books:

- "Cross Currents: The Perils of Electropollution" by Dr. Robert O. Becker.

- "Electromagnetic Fields: A Consumer's Guide to the Issue and How to Protect Ourselves" by B. Blake Levitt.

- "The Invisible Disease: The Dangers of Environmental Illnesses Caused by Electromagnetic Fields and Chemical Emissions" by Gunni Nordstrom.

- "The Force: Living Safely in a World of Electromagnetic Pollution." by Lyn McClean.

- "Silent Fields" and "Dirty Electricity and Electromagnetic Radiation" by Donna Fisher.

Biological defects associated with electromagnetic interference (EMI) can be found in "Light, Radiation, and You." by Dr. John N. Ott.

Human health issues in the electronics industry is well documented in "Challenging the Chip: Labor Rights and Environmental Justice in the Global Electronics Industry." by

Ted Smith, David A. Sonnenfeld, David Naguib Pellow, and Jim Hightower.

I can recommend the free BioInitiative 2012 report for further reading on the subject of wireless radiation:

http://www.bioinitiative.org/

Books that document the known biologically harmful effects of wireless radiation are:

- "Disconnect" by Devra Davis.
- "Public Health SOS: The Shadow Side of the Wireless Revolution" by Magda Havas and Camilla Rees.
- "Cellular Telephone Russian Roulette" by Robert Kane.

Dr. Magda Havas has an excellent electromagnetic website at: www.magdahavas.com

A nice list of research papers about "Dirty Electricity" and the effects on human health can be found at: http://www.stetzerelectric.com/researchPaper/list

Stray voltage reducing products are available and a popular product is the "Ronk Blocker" from Ronk Electrical Industries.

For detecting dirty electricity, Stetzer Electric have developed the "STETZERiZER Meter".

"All the things that human beings suffer from are how their environment treats them, and how the elements of their planet affects their mind and body - like radiation, cancer, and all."

Ornette Coleman

Metals

We cannot live without metals in our food and water. Metals provide the human mind and body the ability to generate DC voltage. Without the DC voltage we would eventually get sick. Metals have a wide range of functions in the biological system of the human and we are only at the start of understanding these processes. Mined and purified metals are the opposite and present a hazard to the human.

The use of metals is a very unnatural activity of the human. Metals are found dispersed in nature. They are generally mined from underground and many processes are used to extract them from the rock that they are part of. Once concentrated into pure metal, their interaction with the natural environment is greatly changed.

Wherever you find pure metals, you will also find very strange magnetic and electromagnetic fields. This is an issue as the human has not evolved in these strange fields. With the advent of electricity, electronics and wireless communications, there are now very strange electromagnetic radiation induced energies flowing in all metals. As such prolonged contact with metals is likely to be toxic to humans.

You should avoid metals in your home and workplace and instead be using wooden furniture where possible. Metal chairs are a bad idea and you should be sitting on wooden chairs. Metal coil mattresses are another item that you should be avoiding. Instead, you should be sleeping on mattresses made out of natural foam materials.

Metal jewelery should be avoided in a wireless radiation society. The worst form of jewelery is anything that is formed into a loop, as it will exhibit the electromagnetic induction effect that should enhance the energy being produced. Examples of these are rings, watches, necklaces, bangles, hoop earrings, and so on. Metal under wired bras and metal interuterine devices (IUD) should be avoided also.

Metal implants of any kind are a bad idea. Metal fillings, bridges, crowns, and implants should be avoided. If you have an accident and they fuse your bones together with metal, you should have the metal removed after you have healed. Hip implants are generally the largest piece of metal that you see in the human. People who have metal implants should be familiar with the symptoms of Electromagnetic Hypersensitivity and should keep their environment free of electromagnetic interference producing products.

Metal hip implants are already getting caught up in class action lawsuits for various reasons. It is only a matter of time before metal implant patients realize that they have an antenna system installed into them that also acts like an electrode of a battery. Metals installed into the body are likely to interfere with the natural DC voltage processes of the body and set up internal battery discharge currents.

"I have every expectation that we will see the following become a recognized human disease in the future: Metal Sickness"

Steven Magee

Altitude

I have a lot of experience with altitude. I spent three years working at approximately 7,775 feet followed by five years at 13,796 feet and three more years at 6,875 feet. Altitude sickness is very real and the effects that it can have on people are diverse. Feeling faint is a common symptom and I have seen people actually faint at altitude.

When I worked in La Palma in the Canary Islands at 7,775 feet, the observatory was significantly above the tree line. The tree line is located at a very definite altitude. Above it, the vegetation significantly changes to low bushy growth of only a couple of feet tall. The trees at the tree line tend to be disfigured and showing stress. This indicates that the biological environment has changed and is biologically harmful to trees. It is likely a solar radiation effect.

The Hawaii observatory was significantly higher at 13,796 feet. It was a barren place with almost no visible life where the observatory was located. Just lots of rocks and cinder! It was far above the tree line. Our blood oxygen levels would be running at 80% of normal up there.

The Arizona observatory at 6,875 feet was below the tree line. However, it appeared to be high enough to cause growth defects in the trees. I remember the trees up there being twisted and disfigured. You could definitely feel the altitude sickness even at this lower elevation.

Altitude sickness is known to occur in most people above 4,900 feet. Aircraft commonly pressurize their cabins to the air pressure found at 6,900 feet to try and prevent these symptoms from occurring. However, some people still report altitude sickness symptoms at this pressure. They are probably the ones that you see holding the sick bags! Nausea is a feature of altitude sickness.

There are very definite symptoms that are associated with the different levels of altitude and Wikipedia states:

- *High altitude 1,500 to 3,500 metres (4,900 to 11,500 ft) - The onset of physiological effects of diminished inspiratory oxygen pressure (PiO2) includes decreased exercise performance and increased ventilation (lower arterial PCO2). Minor impairment exists in arterial oxygen transport (arterial oxygen saturation (SaO2) at least 90%), but arterial PO2 is significantly diminished. Because of the large number of people who ascend rapidly to altitudes between 2,400 and 4,000 m, high-altitude illness is common in this range.*

- *Very high altitude 3,500 to 5,500 metres (11,500 to 18,000 ft) - Maximum SaO2 falls below 90% as the arterial PO2 falls below 60mmHg. Extreme hypoxemia may occur during exercise, during sleep, and in the presence of high altitude pulmonary edema or other acute lung conditions. Severe altitude illness occurs most commonly in this range.*

- *Extreme altitude above 5,500 metres (18,000 ft) - Marked hypoxemia, hypocapnia, and alkalosis are characteristic of extreme altitudes. Progressive deterioration of physiologic function eventually outstrips acclimatization. As a result, no permanent human habitation occurs above 6,000m. A period of acclimatization is necessary when ascending to extreme altitude; abrupt ascent without supplemental oxygen for other than brief exposures invites severe altitude sickness.*

The Hawaii observatory was so high that we used to stop and acclimatize at 9,200 feet, before heading to the peak.

I was lucky enough to have two positions in Hawaii. The first position had me commuting from sea level to 13,796 feet on a daily basis. I would feel lethargic, have a headache, and show stomach problems during the day. In the evening, I just wanted to lay down and recover. I changed my position to the night shift and found that it was much more agreeable to human health. Indeed, it was one of my motivations to move onto the night shift. On nights I would stay on the mountain at 9,200 feet for five nights and commute up to 13,796 feet to work.

One of the things that I do remember that was distinct about working nights at 13,796 feet were the hallucinations. I saw some strange things on top of that mountain! I knew I was hallucinating and it was manageable feature of my job. I found it absolutely fascinating to see the tricks that the human mind could play on me. It was not often that I would have hallucinations, but it generally would occur on my first night on the mountain where my environmental conditions had been greatly changed. Many people report feeling a "presence" when at high altitudes and I frequently experienced this sensation.

Common to all three observatories where I worked was that the long term staff appeared to get leg problems. Some of them would have very strange walks. Indeed, it was like being in the Monty Python's sketch of "The Ministry of Silly Walks"! It was as if their joints had gone stiff. They also did not appear to be very healthy. I suspect that it was caused by daily high altitude commuting and the strange environmental conditions that they were working in. This appears to be called "Delayed Radiation Myelopathy" and is well documented in the medical field of nuclear medicine.

I did see two of the long term full time mountain employees die of disease. These disease conditions that they had were preceded by many years of poor health and both had the strange walks that I was observing. I imagine that high altitude commuting increases the risks of illness, disease and premature death.

This leads me into the purpose of this chapter and that is as you increase in altitude, your environmental conditions significantly change. The higher you go, the greater the change is. There are a wide variety of changes that occur and we will look into these.

Temperature is the most obvious change. The higher you go, the cooler it gets. In Hawaii, you could be sunbathing in shorts on the beach in the morning and by the afternoon you would be in your winter clothes making snowmen on top of the mountain! The temperature change between sea level and 13,796 feet can be extreme.

Less noticeable is the change in solar radiation levels. The sunlight is stronger and has frequencies of radiation in it that you will never find at sea level. As such, the solar radiation conditions are unnatural to the human. We see the effects of this at the tree line in the stressed trees. The ultraviolet levels increase by approximately 10% to 12% with every increase of 3,281 feet in altitude.

If you were to take a Geiger counter to altitude, you would notice that there are far more counts per minute (CPM) on it. This is because the closer you get to Space, the higher the radioactivity from Space becomes! The difference between being below 4,900 feet and above 4,900 feet is significant. Cosmic radiation exposures approximately double with every four thousand feet increase in altitude. This is most certainly an issue for frequent air travelers. At 35 degrees north latitude we find the radiation levels at altitude are:

- **0 Feet = 0.04 micro Sieverts per hour.**
- **10,000 Feet = 0.19 micro Sieverts per hour.**
- **20,000 Feet = 0.99 micro Sieverts per hour.**
- **30,000 Feet = 3.25 micro Sieverts per hour.**
- **40,000 Feet = 6.68 micro Sieverts per hour.**

Nighttime radiation levels are different also. Less atmospheric filtering is taking place and the radiation levels from Space are much higher. You actually see less stars up there, due to the eyes being starved of oxygen. They lose some of their nighttime sensitivity.

Radiation from artificial satellites is greatly increased due to the thinner atmosphere absorbing less artificial radiation. You will be exposed to much higher radio frequencies from the global positioning system (GPS), communication satellites and RADAR mapping satellites. LASER mapping satellites will expose you to higher levels of their radiation. I was a little surprised to find that my cell phone would work at 13,796 feet and it indicates that ground based transmitters are extensively radiating out to Space.

The electrical conductivity of the air is very different. The air at altitude is in a partial vacuum and the density is far less. Nikola Tesla had noted during his research into wireless energy transmission that it was preferable to transmit at altitude due to the better conductivity of air to high electrical frequencies. He states that the conductivity was "*better than copper wire*". This electrical conductivity of the air increases approximately exponentially with altitude.

The air is also electrically charged, as Wikipedia states: *Atmospheric electricity abounds in the environment; some traces of it are found less than four feet from the surface of the earth, but on attaining greater height it becomes more apparent. The main concept is that the air above the surface of the earth is usually, during fine weather, positively electrified, or at least that it is positive with respect to the Earth's surface, the Earth's surface being relatively negative.*

The measurements of atmospheric electricity can be seen as measurements of difference of potential between a point of the Earth's surface, and a point somewhere in the air above it. The atmosphere in different regions is often found to be at different local potentials, which differ from that of the ground sometimes even by as much as 3000 Volts within 100 feet (30 m).

Pressure is less and your body has to work harder to extract oxygen from the thinner air. The body will create extra blood cells and the blood will thicken. Everything in your body will start to expand as the pressure reduces. Your body is constantly working to address these expansion issues. You will need to be drinking plenty of water and electrolytes to enable the body to adapt. The opposite effects occur as you descend to lower elevations. Pressure changes are well known for their ability to make bones ache.

The humidity can either be extremely low if it is clear or extremely high if you are in the clouds.

As you can see, the environment at altitude is very different to what it is at sea level. For the purpose of human health, it appears that it is wise to work and live below 4,900 feet. Living and working above this altitude is likely to lead to altitude related health problems occurring. If you do work at altitude then daily commuting to altitude is undesirable and it is far better to stay there until your work is completed. You should probably not stay in a high altitude job for a long period of time and be aware that you are increasing your risks of illness, disease, cancer, and mental health problems in such jobs. Living or working near or above the tree line is not advisable.

You should only be living and working at altitude if you can trace your genetics to it. People in high cities such as La Paz, Bolivia, at an elevation of 11,942 ft will be genetically adapted to that area. For them, they would be wise to stay at that elevation.

Living at sea level may also be an issue today, particularly in or near to large coastal cities. Much of the pollution that is created by these will stay at sea level. The majority of pollutants are heavier than air and may stay near to the ground as they cool. This can be seen in large cities like Los Angeles as a cloud of pollution hanging over the city. It can also be seen near to erupting volcanoes.

If you live in locations such as these, it is advisable to live at an altitude that puts you above the pollution cloud. The ideal location for human health is not to live in such a polluted area.

"Because of the high altitude, you get drunk really fast. So everyone's drunk all the time."

Clea Duvall

Sounds & Vibrations

With the advent of wind turbines, sound and vibrations have started to receive the attention that they deserve. Extra low frequencies are now produced as part of modern society and they appear to be affecting some of the people that are exposed to them.

It is being widely reported that wind turbines are creating sounds and vibrations that can be sensed by people up to ten miles away! The book "Wind Turbine Syndrome" by Nina Pierpont MD PhD is reporting that people who live within two kilometers of wind turbines are reporting sickness that can be traced to the presence of these.

Dr. Nina Pierpont is reporting that similar symptoms also appear in humans near to natural gas compressor stations, industrial sewage pumping stations, and other power plants. Low frequency noise and infra-sound appear to be the problem.

Wind turbines that have been placed into the ocean will create frequencies and energy in the ocean that may upset the natural life there. It will be interesting to see the effects that these giants have on the long term ocean environment.

Living near busy roads and interstates may cause similar issues. A town that has an air-force base may have jets that go supersonic nearby. If so, you may find silent sonic boom infra-sound waves passing through your property. The supersonic airliner Concorde was famous for creating infra-sound that could be detected 200 miles away!

The Wikipedia article *"United States Navy in Vieques"* states: *In a study...48 of the 50 Vieques residents tested were diagnosed as suffering from vibroacoustic disease — a thickening of heart tissue caused by exposure to sonic booms. This disease is said to lead to heart arrhythmia, or even death.*

These sound waves that are created by modern society are carried on the wind and the direction of the wind will have a large impact on the noise that is created in the local environment daily.

Many people report their symptoms alleviate when they turn off fans in their homes and workplaces. This is because spinning fan blades can fill the surrounding area with infra-sound. I actually found that my air conditioning unit was mounted directly to the attic floor without any anti-vibration mounts. Such a system can induce infra-sound throughout the entire home!

You can easily make an infra-sound detector by opening a large window and placing a flexible sheet of clear acrylic up against the opening. Tack the three sides in place that are next to the frame to make them seal with the window frame. The side of the acrylic that is in the center of the window frame needs to be supported by a metal window screening bar that is flexible enough so that the wind can push the window and flex the acrylic pane. When infra-sound comes through from a supersonic jet or lightning, you will notice that the acrylic window will flex and vibrate.

When choosing a place to live, it makes sense not to be near industrial equipment and main roads. In the case of transportation systems, you will be getting subjected to the chemical pollution that they create also.

"The three great elemental sounds in nature are the sound of rain, the sound of wind in a primeval wood, and the sound of outer ocean on a beach."

Henry Beston

Chemical Exposure

Modern society is filled with chemicals that may be poisoning you. You are exposed to them almost everywhere you go. Here is a list of some of the things that you may want to avoid:

- Soaps.
- Shampoo and conditioners.
- Toothpaste.
- Mouthwash.
- Make up.
- Sunscreen.
- Lipstick.
- Nail varnish.
- Pesticides.
- Herbicides.
- Genetically modified foods.
- Processed foods.
- Medications.
- Exhaust emissions.
- Air fresheners.
- Scented candles.
- Stale air.
- Paint.
- Certain man-made materials.

If it is not natural, then you should be querying whether you should be exposing yourself to it. I recommend that you use organic versions of products where possible.

Many chemicals can cause photo-sensitivity to occur, as they can react with Sunlight. This can mislead you into thinking that you are allergic to the Sun. If you are having reactions to the Sun and you are sure that you are not sunlight deficient, then you should start to examine the chemicals on both the inside and outside of your body. These chemicals may be coming into you from the food and drinks that you are ingesting, and perhaps the air that you are breathing if you are near to air pollution.

Probably the only thing that should come into contact with your skin is natural clothing, natural materials (such as wood) and water. Avoid contact with plastics, synthetic fibers, metals, electronics, chemicals, soaps, make-up, and so on.

Multiple Chemical Sensitivity (MCS) is an emerging illness in the population and is caused by excessive exposure to chemicals. The documentary film "The Tomato Effect" by Faun Kime does a good job of explaining MCS and the corporate denials of its existence.

"You should keep human contact with man-made chemicals to a minimum."

Steven Magee

Society

"When machines and computers, profit motives and property rights are considered more important than people, the giant triplets of racism, materialism, and militarism are incapable of being conquered."
Martin Luther King

The society that you are born into can have major implications for your health. If you are born into a polluted industrial town, it is reasonable to expect that you will have illness in your childhood development that may linger with you for the rest of your life. If you are born into a natural rural environment with little modern development, then you will probably develop with few problems on the way to adulthood.

The more a society changes the natural environment to an industrialized environment then the more health problems that this will cause. Some of the problems that developing a natural environment with modern construction techniques can bring are:

- Loss of tree canopy.
- Loss or reduction of atmospheric DC voltage.
- Increased solar radiation power levels.
- Loss of nature modified solar radiation.
- Loss of ground vegetation.
- Loss of wild animal habitat and ecological systems.
- Loss of natural smells.
- Loss of natural pollen levels.
- Loss of natural sources of water.
- Loss of natural sources of food.

- Pollution.

- Crime.

- Lower quality of general health.

- Increased illness.

- Shorter or longer lifespan, depending on the pollution that you have been exposed to.

- The many man-made diseases of modern society:
  - Allergies.
  - Obesity.
  - Leukemia.
  - Diabetes.
  - Organ failure.
  - Cancer.
  - Aggression.
  - Depression.
  - Dementia.
  - Mental illness.
  - Electromagnetic Hypersensitivity (EHS).
  - Multiple Chemical Sensitivity (MCS).

Of course, no government official will ever tell you that the cities may be making the people in them ill. Nor will they tell you which professions have the shortest lifespans, increased rates of depression, or the highest illness, disease, cancer, and mental illness rates.

Talking about lifespans, some of the professions that appear to have poorer health and shorter lifespans than most are:

- Military.

- Police officer.

- Electrical line worker.

- Electrical switch yard worker.

- Communications field engineer.

- Power inverter field engineer.

- Pilot.

- Welder.

The next chart lists the most common professions for high rates of occupational deaths. When choosing a career, you should pay attention to statistics such as these.

Selected occupations with high fatality rates, 2006

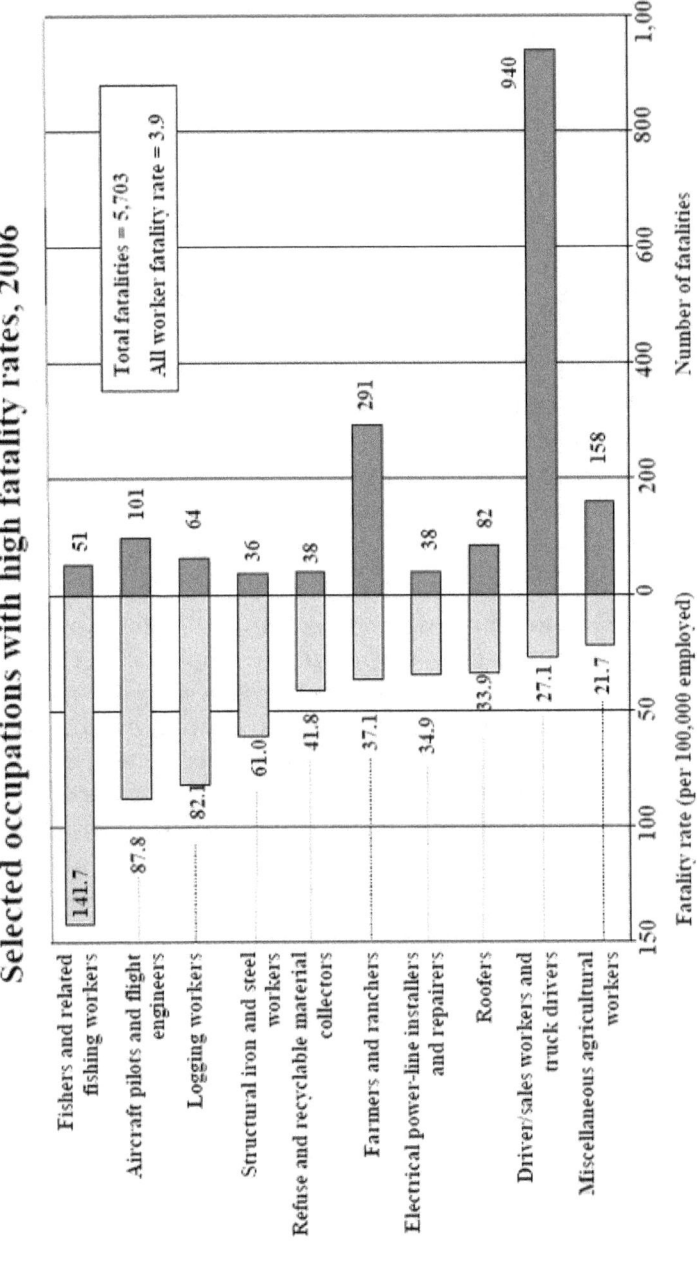

Total fatalities = 5,703
All worker fatality rate = 3.9

It is interesting to note that for police officers, there is a well known observation of them which is called "Angry Aggression Theory"! As applied to police behavior, angry aggression theory argues that the chronic stress of police work along with the inability to respond to the actual sources of that stress increase both the perception of threats and the aggressiveness of responses to perceived threats. So what could be causing "Angry Aggression" in police officers? If you look at the above list you will see that they all have one thing in common: They all work in high electromagnetic radiation environments!

Dr. John Nash Ott proved the link between human health and electromagnetic interference (EMI) back in the 1950's in his book "My Ivory Cellar". Unfortunately, much of his work has been ignored, despite his attempts to get the government to research this area. It is of interest that although on the surface the government ignored the majority of Dr. John Nash Ott's work, they did go on to develop war weapons for the military that use EMI to inflict pain on the human body.

The cure for cancer will go down in history as the biggest government and corporate cover-up ever! As a result of Dr. John Nash Ott's work, cancer was well understood back in the 1950's and the covering up of both the cause and the cure for cancer has been part of the corporate and government culture since then. As Adrienne Rich says *"Lying is done with words and also with silence."* This silence is well documented in the book "The Secret History of the War on Cancer" by Devra Davis.

Time is one of the products of modern human society. When you examine time and how it relates to the cycles of nature, it appears to be a very flawed human concept. Most people are now working a forty hour week with ten days of vacation in the USA. The day starts at 8am and finishes at 5pm, Monday through to Friday. They are probably working in an office with electronic florescent lighting, computers, air conditioning, and energy star glass and, as such, they may be quite ill!

The problem with this is that the human mind and body does not function this way. The human mind and body is actually tied into the sunrise and the sunset for waking and sleeping. Therefore, in winter you may actually find yourself going to work in the dark and coming home in the dark! A very interesting concept for a creature that is not supposed to be awake before sunrise and should go to bed at sunset.

It is also a problem when it comes to the photosynthesis effects that take place within the human mind and body. If you are not exposing yourself to sunlight throughout the week then you may go into sunlight withdrawal. There are many people in modern society that are in some level of sunlight withdrawal and they do not realize it. It is commonly documented as Seasonal Affect Disorder (SAD) and causes a wide range of symptoms to appear during wintertime.

The really interesting thing is that there are many people who are in sunlight deficiency in the summertime! This can occur if you spend very little time outside during the week. In modern society this is a relatively easy state to fall into with the use of cars, homes, offices and indoor shopping. Walking to work or to the shops is becoming a thing of the past.

It is proposed that the correct work environment for the human should start no earlier than two hours after sunrise and finish no later than two hours before sunset. This would allow the human to revert back to its natural state of following the solar cycles for sleeping and waking periods.

The human addiction of using large amounts of energy to move humans and goods around should be stopped. A car is incredibly heavy and has a very inefficient engine. When you look at most people's jobs, they could easily be done from home. In an era of dwindling resources, one can only wonder about a society that requires its workers to commute daily to work by collectively burning massive amounts of fossil fuels. We should be moving towards a society that is local based in every aspect. Transportation of people and goods should be seen as a last resort and not the norm.

Toxic Health © Steven Magee

This use of fossil fuels is driven by governments that are heavily influenced by corporations. In the world of modern business and stock markets, a corporations success is determined by its profits. For corporations to make more profits, they need people to consume more. The modern governments encourage consumption to ensure that the corporations that fund their election campaigns continue to do so! It has been noticed by many that corporate donations and the corporate lobbying of the government has led to an arguably corrupt political system that works against the people and not for them.

A facet of this corruption is evidenced in the control of information to the masses. The mainstream media is now under the control of the corporations and they will select the information that is to be presented to the masses. Government media sources appear to be behaving in a similar fashion. An example of this was when the Fukushima nuclear power plant was venting radioactive steam into the environment in 2011 and the media was describing it as a *"harmless release of radiation"*! Who has ever heard of such a thing? The Fukushima nuclear complex went on to become the worst man-made engineering disaster in all of human history, outside of war.

Delivery of public information is now somewhat corrupted and once you become aware of this, it becomes hard to believe the information that is presented daily to the masses as "News". An example of this was the opening of Hoover Dam in the USA. Opened by the President of the USA as a wonderful achievement, in actuality, mistakes had been made in the construction of the project and it was quietly fixed over the following decade under a veil of secrecy. There have been many books written about the government's addiction to secrecy from their own people and "Secrets and Lies" by David Southwell is a good example of this. In 2011 the United States of America's Defense Secretary, Robert Gates, openly admitted that most governments lie.

As L. Neil Smith says *"I'm tired of being lied to by government, by the media, and by every corporation I have anything to do with."*

Wars have been prevalent in the last century and this should come as no surprise to those who understand the natural world. The modern human has destroyed its natural environment and created an extremely high man-made electromagnetic environment and a heavily polluted environment in general that creates corruption and aggression. Two-time Congressional Medal of Honor winner Maj. Gen. Smedley Butler had it right 75 years ago when he said of war: *"It is possibly the oldest, easily the most profitable, surely the most vicious [racket]...It is the only one in which the profits are reckoned in dollars and the losses in lives...It is conducted for the benefit of the very few, at the expense of the very many."*

There appears to have been a distortion of the truth regarding terrorism in the modern world. UNC sociology professor Charles Kurzman specializes in Middle East and Islamic studies, but he knows his American history too. *"Muslims are the latest wave of immigrants who are associated with acts of violence and are thought to be disloyal or not fully American, who are thought by many people to be impossible to integrate into American society. It was the same for the Irish in the 1840s, for Germans from the 1860s through World War I and for Italians who early in 20th Century were associated with anarchism and socialism and for Japanese Americans after Pearl Harbor,"* Kurzman said. Much of Kurzman's recent work has been to compile statistical profiles of Muslim Americans that reveal the majority of Muslim Americans are not the demons that some politicians and pundits have made them appear after 9-11.

Professor William Odom, formerly President Reagan's NSA Director wrote: *"As many critics have pointed, out, terrorism is not an enemy. It is a tactic. Because the United States itself has a long record of supporting terrorists and using terrorist tactics, the slogans of today's war on terrorism merely makes the United States look hypocritical to the rest of the world."*

The cost of the 9-11 attacks through to the Bin Laden assassination is estimated at 3 trillion dollars, the United States of America is heavily in debt, unemployment is high and many large corporations do not pay taxes. It is clear that something has gone wrong in the government system! Martin Luther King had it right when he said *"Our scientific power has outrun our spiritual power. We have guided missiles and misguided men."*

The history that is now being taught to many school children is somewhat distorted. The government writes and carefully selects the information that children are to be taught from and one can only wonder why the events are not entirely accurately portrayed in the history books that they use. There are many books that discuss this concept and "Lies My Teacher Told Me: Everything Your American History Textbook Got Wrong." by James W. Loewen is one example of this.

Children are now raised to "get a job" instead of enjoying childhood. If we look at traditional rural cultures, children are raised by their families through to adulthood. School does not exist and the teaching is from father to son. What child really aspires to go to school and get a job? Most children I know want to spend time with their families and friends. Being educated by strangers in a school that is miles away from their home is generally not high in their priorities. Separating children from their families in an effort to educate them for incorporation into an industrial machine is a flawed social policy.

Capitalism has shown its true colors in the energy industry. Labeling toxic processes as "clean and green", such as coal, gas, and nuclear energy is a very clear case of "Green-washing". It is clearly not true! The energy industry branding itself as clean and green is possibly one of the biggest lies ever told to the population. The lie is needed to keep the Industrial Revolution going at the expense of the mass population, nature and ultimately, the Earth. Capitalism appears to be following a policy of lie, confuse and deny in order to keep economic expansion progressing. As Upton Sinclair observed *"It is difficult to get a man to understand something when his job depends on not understanding it."*

It appears that capitalism has reached the lose-lose situation. The continued expansion of the destruction of natural systems to provide for the consumption for an ever increasing world population will lead to human extinction as

the natural systems become more polluted. They will all start to shut down, leaving humanity stranded with no further options. As Gandhi said *"The Earth provides enough to satisfy every man's need, but not every man's greed."*

Future historians will regard the era of capitalism as a disease of an insane mind. Unfortunately, the modern human is so badly polluted from the destruction of its own environment that it thinks the current situation is completely normal!

The longer climate change is ignored by modern governments and ineffective policies are followed, the bigger the task of effective change becomes. Lester R. Brown has recognized this in his book "Plan B 4.0: Mobilizing to Save Civilization". Change could have been easily effected back in the 1950's by governments to prevent the situation that we find ourselves in today. As each year passes, little changes and everything becomes more polluted. It is clear that continued expansion and pollution is a path to the collective suicide of humanity. At the point where the mass population realizes exactly how serious the situation is, it will require more effort than all of the wars put together to effect change, assuming that it is not too late to change at that time.

Reform for the people and by the people is required to prevent humanity from pursuing the path to extinction. A switch from focusing on profits to that of the future generation's inheritance is needed, as we are the keepers of the Earth. I am personally ashamed of the inheritance that has been left by my generation. The next generation has a huge task ahead of them.

The following books would be good further reading on this subject:

- "Why Leaders Lie: The Truth About Lying in International Politics." by John J. Mearsheimer.
- "Political Ponerology: A Science on the Nature of Evil Adjusted for Political Purposes." by Andrzej M. Lobaczewski.

- "Denialism: How Irrational Thinking Harms the Planet and Threatens our Lives." by Michael Specter.

- "Sparking a Worldwide Energy Revolution: Social Struggles in the Transition to a Post Petrol World." by Kolya Abramsky.

- "The Transition Handbook: From Oil Dependancy to Local Resilience." by Rob Hopkins.

"The price good men pay for indifference to public affairs is to be ruled by evil men."

Plato

Radiation Detoxification

Can you detoxify from radiation? Yes you can! The radiation detoxification can be very painful and extended. It may take several months to go through the first detoxification and it will vary with the individual and how polluted they are. You should be under medical guidance and supervision if you choose to do this.

The human body is like a bucket that is constantly filling up with toxins. If the toxic exposures are too high, then those toxins will start to overwhelm the human body. If the toxin level rises quickly, you will get very sick and may go on to develop disease in a short period of time. If the toxin level is rising slowly, then you will slowly get sick and may go on to develop disease over a much longer time period.

Generally, this time period will be years, or even decades. When you examine the human death statistics, you see that the death rate starts rising significantly after the age of thirty and this is when most people start reporting health problems. It appears that many people have become really toxic by the age of thirty!

The only known way to empty out the toxins from the human body is to detoxify.

The human "Toxic Bucket" is shown on the next page.

Toxic Bucket

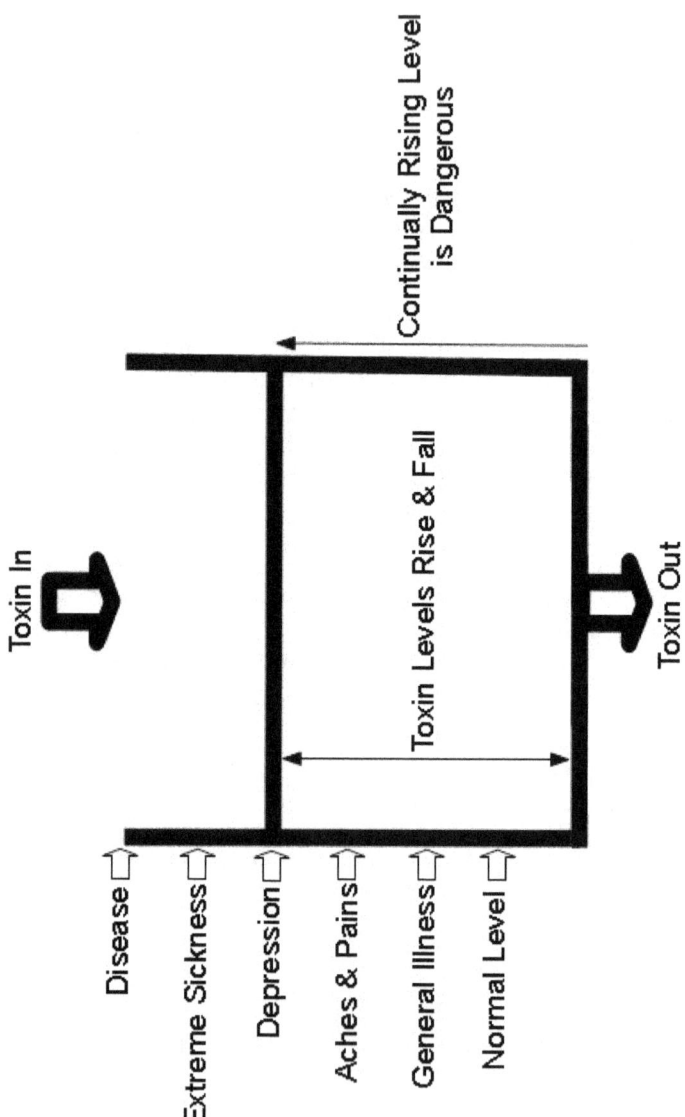

Here are the steps that I developed for the radiation detoxification:

- Switch off all but essential electrical circuits at the fuse board.

- Switch off all but essential electrical and electronic items in your home.

- Take all wireless radiation producing equipment out of service.

- Change all electric lighting to filament light bulbs.

- Artificial lighting should be minimal and just sufficient for the task.

- Cover all windows with window coverings.

- Your home lighting level should be very low both in the day and the night.

- Do not spend time near the windows or in bright parts of your home.

- Stay covered up with clothing when indoors so that you do not absorb light.

- Keep skin exposure to outdoor light minimal by covering up as much as possible when outside.

- Use dark, neutral density sunglasses and wide brimmed hats when outside.

- Do not use sunscreen, make-up, lipstick, or have painted nails.

- Avoid using products such as toothpaste, shampoo, soap, and so on during this process. Shower, bathe, and clean your teeth with water only.

- Eat fresh organic food.

- Drink mineral water.

- Go to bed at sunset and wake up at sunrise.

- It is preferable to stay in bed as long as possible each day in a dark room.

- Your bedroom should be completely dark at night.

The detoxification can be severe in the first month with flu-like symptoms as you withdraw from natural radiation and artificial radiation exposures. You may see heart arrhythmia problems during the detoxification and this appears to be a normal part of the process.

Fatigue follows for a few months and this can be severe. It gradually gets better the longer you are detoxing. I would recommend that you detoxify for no more than three months at a time. If you detoxify for too long you may go into vitamin D and B12 deficiency, and extreme fatigue may appear. You will know when you are in sunlight deficiency as you will start to get headaches that match the changing levels of light exposure from being near windows for too long. You will get very anxious with rapid heartbeats, tight vocal cords, and difficulty breathing when placed into stressful situations. If you get to this point, then it is time to stop detoxing and to slowly return to daylight exposure.

Once detoxing is completed, gradually increase your solar radiation exposure to a few hours per day in the shade of trees over several weeks. Obtaining solar radiation in the shade of trees appears to be important in human health due to the modification of solar radiation that takes place in the tree canopy. I recommend starting with 5 minutes in the morning on your first day and increasing by a further 5 minutes each day until you reach your normal daylight exposure level.

The human mind and body can go into solar radiation overload if you spend too much time outdoors and you will need to figure out where the correct solar radiation exposure time is for you by experimentation. Your pain system will let you know if you get too much exposure to solar radiation. Some of this overload appears to come from exposure to the wireless radiation that we are now immersed into and it is preferable to avoid known high wireless radiation environments. Avoid obtaining outdoor exposures in areas with cell phone towers, TV and radio transmitters, government buildings, ports, airports, military bases, hospitals, transmitting utility meters, and so on.

The good news is that after detoxing from radiation exposure, you should feel like a young person again and be free from aches and pains. It is worth the trouble to move into good health.

After the first detox, you should detox in the middle of winter for forty days and nights each year. The detox appears necessary for good human health. After you are detoxed, you will start to realize exactly how much pollution you are being exposed to, as you will feel the effects of it.

I developed the radiation detoxification process in 2010 with a six month long detoxification that was extremely severe. My second detoxification was a 40 day long process that was much milder and I attribute that to avoiding electromagnetic radiation and high solar radiation exposures during the year.

My third detoxification was extremely mild and short at just two weeks of staying indoors and avoiding daylight. I only saw mild heart arrhythmia occur during it. The purpose of the short detoxification was to see how my body would react to a rapid introduction back to sunlight. This is what I found:

Day 1 – 15 minutes late afternoon sunlight exposure.

Day 2 – 30 minutes late afternoon sunlight exposure.

Day 3 – 45 minutes late afternoon sunlight exposure.

Day 4 – 1 hour late afternoon sunlight exposure.

Each night I had really bad insomnia and my sleep cycle kicked in at sunrise! Every evening I had headaches that occurred a few hours after the exposure to sunlight. The headaches would not respond to Ibuprofen. During the daytime I was fatigued due to lack of sleep.

I changed the process over the next few days due to a trip that I had planned:

Day 5 – Pulled up the window blinds on my home to make the house bright. Spent 1 hour outside near to sunset. I had a bunged up and runny nose.

Day 6 – 3 hours of afternoon driving north in bright winter sunlight in Southern Arizona.

Day 7 - 3 hours of afternoon driving south in bright winter sunlight in Southern Arizona.

The headaches and fatigue subsided during this time, but the insomnia continued.

I changed the sunlight schedule again to eliminate the insomnia:

Day 8, 9, 10, 11 – Window blinds up all day with half hour sunlight exposure near sunset.

The insomnia cleared up but was replaced by fatigue. I changed the outdoor schedule to 2 hours of afternoon walks. This schedule reinstated my normal health pattern after approximately one week.

I realized during this process that a rapid introduction to sunlight is not advisable and you should adjust your outdoor exposures to avoid producing headaches and insomnia. Both are undesirable. If adverse symptoms show up, then simply reduce your solar radiation exposure levels until they clear up before continuing to increase outdoor exposures back to normal levels. You may have to adjust your exposure levels several times during the process to complete a smooth return to normal solar radiation levels. Mid morning sunlight exposures appear to be far better than afternoon exposures and avoid exposures within an hour of sunrise or sunset due to the low ultraviolet content.

As you can see, a rapid introduction to sunlight still will take time. There appears to be a limit as to how fast you can do it without triggering adverse health symptoms. You should schedule a radiation detoxification with ample time for the hibernation period and also the recovery period. It is a bad idea to be time constrained when using this health technique.

After the detoxification process, exposure to electromagnetic fields is one of the things that will become very noticeable to you. You will feel like you are allergic to it, due to the reactions that your body will have to it.

This leads me to the conclusion that the reason why people are allergic to pollen is that they have withdrawn too much from nature. The same thing happens with the Sun if you avoid it, you will become "allergic" to it! The only way to start to feel good around things that you are "allergic" to is to continually expose yourself to it so that your body becomes used to the presence of it. It is the same for electromagnetic radiation. Unfortunately, unlike pollen and sunlight, man-made electromagnetic radiation is likely to do long-term damage to your health!

"The radiation detoxification process exists in nature. It is called: Hibernation."

Steven Magee

Aggression

When reviewing the 2013 myfoxny.com article *America's anger epidemic: why?* we find that *A recent study from the USA Today found 60 percent of Americans report feeling angry or irritable. That is up from 50 percent when a similar poll was taken in 2011.* Suicides are also on the rise in the USA and young people are shooting up their schools.

Why is this occurring? Humans have already started to figure out that nature is essential to good mental and physical health, as this United States Department of Agriculture article demonstrates:

Do Trees Strengthen Urban Communities, Reduce Domestic Violence? By W. C. Sullivan, Ph.D. & Frances E. Kuo, Ph.D.

Cities are characterized by a whole host of social ills-- from anonymity, to incivility, to outright violence--that are strikingly less prevalent in rural areas. Why is this? The physical environment a person lives in has profound effects on their social behavior. Social psychologists have shown that people in cities behave differently from people in rural areas in part because they live in crowded, noisy places, or in places that lack open space. But cities differ from rural areas in another important way as well--rural areas have something that's often lacking in urban areas--nature. Can part of the unsociableness of city dwellers be traced to the lack of plants in their everyday surroundings?

With support from the National Urban Community Forestry Advisory Council, we set out to answer these questions in one of the grimmest of urban settings--public housing in a major city.

As these pictures show, the number of trees immediately outside each of the 28 buildings at Robert Taylor Homes in Chicago vary considerably. Some buildings are surrounded only by concrete and asphalt, while others have trees, grass, and even

250

flowers. Using aerial photographs and on-site analyses we chose 10 buildings with trees and 8 buildings without trees. We then interviewed 75 African-American women living in those buildings about their social behavior and compared the answers from women living in different buildings.

While the amount of plant life varies from building to building, very little else does. The buildings are architecturally identical. There are no systematic differences in the groups of people living in one building or another, perhaps because residents have very little choice in the specific apartment they are assigned. This gives us some confidence that differences we find in social behavior of people living in buildings with and without trees are really due to the trees--not differences in crowding, noise levels, or availability of open space, not differences in race, economic status, or even nature preferences in the people living there.

Do people who live in buildings with trees get along and treat each other better than people living in buildings without trees? The results of these interviews are not only interesting; they also provide new arguments in support of urban forest programs. Let's look at some of the highlights.

DO TREES STRENGTHEN URBAN COMMUNITIES?

For some time there have been stories about community gardens revitalizing inner city urban neighborhoods (Francis, Cashdan & Paxson 1984; Lewis 1972, 1979). Until now, however, no one has systematically examined the effect of trees on relations among neighbors.

We are finding signs of stronger communities where there are trees. In buildings with trees, people report significantly better relations with their neighbors. In buildings without trees, people report having fewer visitors and knowing fewer people in the building. In buildings with trees, people report a stronger feeling of unity and cohesion with their neighbors; they like where they are living more and they feel safer than residents who have few trees around them.

Why might trees contribute to better relations among neighbors? In 100 observations of outdoor common spaces in two public housing developments, we are finding that outdoor spaces with trees are used significantly more often than identical spaces without trees. We suspect that in urban areas, trees create outdoor spaces that attract people. When people are drawn to spaces with trees, they are more likely to see and interact with their neighbors, more likely to get to know each other and become friends.

Stronger ties among neighbors may be a good thing, but it becomes an even more convincing reason to support urban forests when you consider what neighborhood ties mean for residents' functioning. There is evidence that people with strong neighborhood ties are more physically healthy (Cassel 1976; Cobb 1976), more mentally healthy (Gottlieb 1983), less likely to neglect or abuse their children (Garbarino & Sherman 1980), and less likely to rely on costly social services in times of need (Biegel 1994; Gottlieb 1983; Collins & Pancoast 1976). In other words, these findings suggest that by investing in urban forests, a city might reap such dividends as a lowered incidence of child abuse, and decreased demand on social services.

DO TREES REDUCE VIOLENCE?

Two studies have shown a connection between trees and lower levels of violence (Mooney & Nicell 1992; Rice & Remy, in press). But these studies involved prison inmates, and Alzheimer patients living in nursing homes. What about people who are not living in institutional settings?

We are finding less violence in urban public housing where there are trees. Residents from buildings with trees report using more constructive, less violent ways of dealing with conflict in their homes. They report using reasoning more often in conflicts with their children, and they report significantly less use of severe violence. And in conflicts with their partners, they report less use of physical violence than do residents living in buildings without trees.

Why might trees contribute to less violence in the home? Imagine feeling irritated, impulsive, about ready to snap due to the difficulties of living in severe poverty. Having neighbors who you can call on for support means you have an alternative way of dealing with your frustrations other than striking out against someone. Places with nature and trees may provide settings in which relationships grow stronger and violence is reduced.

WHAT DOES THIS MEAN FOR URBAN FORESTRY?

In times of tight budgets, public officials look to reduce costs, and in doing so it is reasonable that they eliminate amenities. Trees have often been considered amenities. But what if urban foresters could report to city officials that trees help lower social service budgets, decrease police calls for domestic violence, strengthen urban communities, and decrease the incidence of child abuse in a city? Would the urban forest be considered an amenity then?

In this study, we are finding that urban forests help build stronger communities, and in doing so, they contribute to lower levels of domestic violence. Although no strong conclusions can be made from a single study, these findings are encouraging and exciting. At a time when the nation's attention is focused on issues such as crime prevention, health care, and the plight of single mothers, these findings suggest that trees can help address some of the most important problems in society today. We believe that urban forests are not mere amenities--that they are a basic part of the infrastructure of any city, as necessary as streets, sewers, and electricity.

REFERENCES

- *Biegel, D.E. (1994). Help seeking and receiving in urban ethnic neighborhoods: strategies for empowerment. Prevention in Human Services. 3 (2-3): 119-143.*

- *Cassel, J. 1976. The contribution of the social environment to host resistance. American Journal of Epidemiology. 104(2): 107-123.*

- *Cobb, S. 1976. Social support as a moderator of life stress. Psychosomatic Medicine. 38(5): 300-314.*

- *Collins, A.H.; Pancoast, D.L. 1976. Natural helping networks: a strategy for prevention. Washington, DC: National Association of Social Workers.*

- *Francis, M.; Cashdan, L.; Paxson, L. 1984. Community open spaces: greening neighborhoods through community action and land conservation. Washington, DC: Island Press.*

- *Garbarino, J.; Sherman, D.1980. High-risk neighborhoods and high-risk families: the human ecology of child maltreatment. Child Development, 51(1): 188-198.*

- *Gottlieb, B.H. 1983. Social support as a focus for integrative research in psychology. American Psychologist. 38(3). 278-285.*

- *Lewis, C.A. 1972. Public housing gardens: landscapes for the soul. In Landscape for Living. Washington DC: United States Department of Agriculture Yearbook of Agriculture.*

- *Leuis, C.A. 1979. The sprouting of the inner city. Psychology Today. 13(1): 12-13.*

- *Mooney, P.; Nicell, P.L. 1992. The importance of exterior environment for Alzheimer residents: effective care and risk management. Gestion des soins de sante. Health Care Management forum: 5(2): 23-29.*

- *Rice, J.S.; Remy; L.L. (in press). Cultivating self development in urban jail inmates. Journal of Offender Rehabilitation.*

Copies of this article and many others on human health and its relation to the trees can be obtained from the Landscape and Human Health Laboratory at the University of Illinois: http://lhhl.illinois.edu/

What is it that could be causing this aggression effect? It is not just one thing, there are multiple things taking place that cause the aggression effect. They can all be summed up by one word:

Pollution

Pollution of the human mind and body takes on many forms and some of them are listed below:

- Unnatural solar radiation spectrum.
- Unnatural solar radiation power levels.
- Solar radiation interference effects.
- Sunlight deficiency.
- Artificial light.
- Exposure to electricity.
- Exposure to electrical, electronic and wireless products.
- Exposure to electromagnetic interference (EMI).
- Exposure to man-made radiation.
- Reduction or loss of atmospheric DC voltage.
- Eating unnatural food.
- Breathing unnatural air.
- Exposure to unnatural smells.
- Pollen deficiency.
- Exposure to unnatural temperatures.
- Drinking unnatural water.
- Exposure to unnatural noise and vibrations.
- Exposure to chemicals.
- Exposure to a poor social society.
- Nature deficiency.

The many sources of pollution are poisoning people in large numbers. My research is indicating that by removing the source of the pollution that is affecting people, their mental and physical health may fully recover to enable them to live a normal and healthy life. If it is not removed, then they will continue with their slowly deteriorating health. Prescription drugs will just mask the underlying problems.

"Your environment defines you."

Steven Magee

Sixth Sense

The sixth human sense is that of pain. It is the alarm system of the human body. To ignore it is like committing suicide. You will only get worse, not better. Humans have invented the pharmaceutical industry to override this system of pain so that humans can keep working, instead of recovering at home. Do not ignore pain!

Many people get general aches and pains. These people had been labeled as hypochondriacs by the medical profession. We now know that the medical profession may be wrong and that most people with general aches and pains are perhaps suffering from the effects of poisoning, most likely electromagnetic interference and solar radiation poisoning.

Do not ignore your pains, they are very real. You need to take action and locate the source of the problem in your environment and remove it to return to good health. A prescription to override it will most likely send you to an early grave.

"There is a saying in the medical profession 'Inside every tablet is a little bit of poison'. Avoid medications if you can."

Steven Magee

Modern Business

Modern business is built on the methodology of constant expansion, profits and increasing human consumption. This strategy does not work on a planet that is made of finite resources. Unfortunately, it appears that the majority of business schools are still teaching this practice, which appears to be severely flawed today.

Business is heavily focused on the masses who now live in the cities. The cities are unnatural man-made environments. A characteristic of the cities are high levels of pollution that include high levels of solar radiation. Pollution is detrimental to human health and may induce illness and disease into the human mind and body.

Business should move to a new model that is likely to be focused on:

- Local production.
- Minimal energy use.
- Energy use from bio-fuels that were locally grown.
- Use of only surface obtained produce and products.
- Minimal transportation.
- A move away from city life.
- A return to rural living under a tree canopy.
- A return to harmony between humans and the natural world.
- A return to a population size that can be easily supported by the natural surface resources of the planet.
- A return to local community life.

If we do not make the changes quickly, what can we expect?

- Unnatural levels of solar radiation.
- A widespread drought.
- Massive localized flooding.
- Global weather extremes.
- A hot atmosphere.
- Water vapor that remains trapped in the hot atmosphere.
- Widespread illness and disease in the world population.
- A possible extinction of many world species of animals and plants.
- A possible human extinction.
- A possible thermal runaway that wipes out the majority of life on the entire planet.
- A sterile planet.

"The biggest threats to human survival today are not wars or conflict, it is modern business."

Steven Magee

Human Environment

We have established that the majority of humans are living in the incorrect environments. So what is the correct environment?

Historians indicate that the humans started out in the tropics in Africa. The tropics in Africa is a lush forested environment with a tree canopy. The tropics has a stable year round climate. They were walking barefoot under the tree canopy, as they would have been burned by the Sun without clothes in the open.

Science has proven that the trees and plants reduce and modify the radiation levels to make them healthy to humans. Eating organic fruits and vegetables is known to prevent free radicals from occurring inside the human body and keeps the body young.

At this point we have our answer. The human environment is supposed to have the following characteristics:

- Tropical.
- Tree canopy.
- Atmospheric DC voltage.
- Uncontaminated ground.
- Tree interference solar radiation.
- Low solar radiation power levels.
- Lots of vegetation.
- Stable, year round, warm temperatures.
- A source of natural surface water.
- A source of natural food.

- No sources of man-made electromagnetic interference (EMI).

To move away from this type of environment is likely to induce pain, illness, and disease into the human mind and body. This has been demonstrated by the high amounts of it in modern society.

Humans can be found in every climate zone on the Earth. They are the only animal that has complete climate zone coverage. The rest of the animals stay within their genetic climate zones, as they know they will get ill outside of them.

Could you imagine a polar bear at the Equator or a pink flamingo at the North Pole? They would surely die in these locations. It is strange that humans cannot see this effect in their own species.

So your health and that of your family and children is important to you, what can you do about this? The answer is quite simple:

- Move to the tropics, preferably the equator.

- Live in an environment that has a tree canopy.

- Follow the solar cycles for waking and sleeping.

- Walk barefoot on uncontaminated ground.

- Eat fresh nourishing food that is grown in a natural way.

- Drink the water from the streams.

- Do not live near to a large city.

- Do not do anything that is unnatural.

- Avoid man-made materials, especially ones derived from fossil fuels.

"A healthy attitude is contagious but don't wait to catch it from others, be a carrier"

Tom Stoppard

Home Selection

Here are some hints and tips for selecting natural electromagnetic radiation homes:

Avoid homes that:

- Are multiple story due to uneven heating and cooling between the different floors, and electrical cables running underneath the upper story floors.
- Have air conditioning units outside of the bedrooms, the noise will keep you awake.
- Are on curves in the road due to lensing effects that reflections from multiple homes may create.
- Are painted in light reflective colors.
- Have smooth exterior walls.
- Have lots of glass.
- Have glass windows that change the color of the light.
- Have pitched roofs that can be seen from the ground.
- Are paved with modern reflective construction materials.
- Are overlooked by taller structures.
- Have views of the roofs of the surrounding homes.
- Have streetlights nearby.
- Are near built up areas, especially industrial zones.
- Are near to utility equipment.
- Are near to transmitter systems.
- Have radiation transmitting utility meters.
- Are devoid of natural wildlife.
- Have no trees or vegetation.

- Have plants and trees that are showing stress.

Look for homes that:
- Are surrounded by trees.
- Have plenty of vegetation.
- Have lots of shade.
- Are covered in climbing plants.
- In a natural setting.
- Are single story only.
- Are old and have aged.
- Are made of natural rough materials such as wood and dark stone.
- Are painted in dark non-reflective colors on the outside.
- Have the majority of windows facing the pole.
- Have "full spectrum" acrylic windows installed.
- Have window coverings on both the inside and outside of the home.
- Have bedrooms facing the pole.
- Have underground utilities.
- Have plenty of distance between the neighboring properties in all directions, preferably several hundred feet.
- Are set back from the street.
- Have housing associations that have banned wireless products and amateur radio operators.

For information on healthy buildings, the free film "First Earth" at http://www.davidsheen.com/firstearth/film.htm provides excellent advice.

"Nature is my manifestation of God. I go to nature every day for inspiration in the day's work. I follow in building the principles which nature has used in its domain."

Frank Lloyd Wright

Toxic Health © Steven Magee

RWS & EHS

Radio Wave Sickness (RWS) and Electromagnetic Hypersensitivity (EHS) are rapidly accelerating plagues in modern society. Sweden appears to be the only country that currently recognizes the conditions. In Sweden approximately 300,000 people are registered as having EHS. Sweden has a population of 9,555,893 as reported in the 2012 census. This equates to 3.12 percent of the population, or 1 in 32 people, that is aware that it is being affected by unnatural radiation exposures which include electrical, electronic and wireless systems.

Elizabeth Kelley MD, Director of the Electromagnetic Safety Alliance, reports that, since the early 1990s, health practitioners world-wide have seen a rapid increase in the number of people who report a cluster of neurological symptoms that is called electromagnetic hypersensitivity. EHS symptoms commonly include headache, sleep problems, poor memory and concentration, depression, anxiety, changes in heart rate and, skin burning sensations. These symptoms are being reported mainly by people who live in the developed world where there has been rapid human adaptation to wireless digital technologies over the past two decades.

In 2005, the World Health Organization published Fact Sheet No 296 entitled Electromagnetic Hypersensitivity: "Well controlled and conducted double-blind studies have shown that symptoms were not correlated with EMF exposure... The symptoms are certainly real and can vary widely in their severity... Further, EHS is not a medical diagnosis, nor is it clear that it represents a single medical problem."

Dr. Olle Johannsson, a Swedish neuroscientist, reports that in Sweden Electrohypersensitivity (EHS) is an officially fully recognized functional impairment and those who have this condition are eligible for government services and accommodations. Recent studies show that over 5% of Swedish men and women report a variety of symptoms when exposed to electromagnetic field (EMF) sources.

Dr. Magda Havas, a professor of environmental science at Trent University in Ontario, Canada, states that EHS studies with negative results can have major biases. "The researchers assumed that reactions to EMFs are immediate, while there is often a delay between exposure and response. People are not switches that can be turned on and off. These studies incorrectly insinuate that, if you can't feel anything, it can't harm you. We know very well that we can't detect the taste of arsenic, lead, DDT nor asbestos, but they are all toxic."

European medical doctors are estimating that, by 2017, 50% of the world's population will be affected by mild to severe EHS symptoms

The problem with RWS and EHS in the USA is that it is commonly misdiagnosed as another condition. The USA has become addicted to wireless communications technologies and electrical and electronic products, so the rates are likely comparable to Sweden. The recent adoption of Smart/AMR/AMI radiation transmitting utility meters in many USA cities has probably significantly increased the number of people who have RWS and EHS, but are currently incorrectly diagnosed.

This is unfortunate, as it is well known today that RWS and EHS is easily preventable. All you have to do is remove the sources of unnatural man-made electromagnetic interference. I find it very concerning that the USA government simply ignores people who are trying to restore their environment back to natural radiation levels in an effort to clear up their RWS and EHS symptoms. It appears to be rare for the Federal Communications Commission (FCC) to enforce rule 15 that relates to harmful electromagnetic interference. Indeed, I recently put rule 15 to the test and notified the FCC that the gas company was causing biologically harmful interference at my home. They simply ignored my request for them to notify the gas company to remove their biologically harmful transmitting meters from the area around my home.

The FCC have established one of the most lax electromagnetic radiation standards in the world. At 61 volts per meter (V/m) for 1800 MHz public exposure, the

permissible radiation emissions are higher than most other countries in the world. For contrast, 0.06 V/m is the recommendation in Salzburg, Austria, which makes the USA standard 1017 times higher! The reason for this ridiculously high standard in the USA is obvious when you look at the military. The most technologically advanced military in the world has been developing wireless warfare for decades. If the FCC was to lower the standards, then they would effectively render some parts of the military arsenal as obsolete.

This same military force who became aware of what RWS and EHS was during the development of RADAR in the 1930's and 1940's appears to have been denying the condition exists from the 1950's onwards! Instead, the opposite happened and electrical, electronic and wireless products were heavily marketed to the masses, while the military who were supposed to protect them from biological harm simply stayed silent.

When you look into how electrical, electronic and wireless products are approved for sale in the USA, you find that no laboratory animals nor plants are used to assess their safety. Instead, electronic meters make measurements and something that resembles Jello is used to assess if the devices can heat it. If the meter readings are within specification and the Jello is not substantially heated, then the product is approved for sale.

The reality is that if these devices were tested on animals and plants, then many of them would fail the tests! As Dr. John Nash Ott discovered in his research that he conducted from the 1950's to the 1980's, many electrical and electronic products change the behaviors of animals and can make them sick, and some of them go on to die premature deaths. He also found that if you subjected an animal to biologically harmful electromagnetic radiation and made it sick, that you could return it to a healthy state simply by removing the harmful exposures. This is exactly what people are reporting who have RWS and EHS!

Dr. John Nash Ott also performed many plant experiments with electromagnetic radiation and he found that plants would react to many common electrical and electronic products. Growth deformities were observed in many of his experiments. I have been able to reproduce much of his work regarding plants and I can tell you that his findings are easily repeatable.

Many government agencies are aware of not only Dr. John Nash Ott's work, but also of the work done by many other researchers. Indeed, I have mailed many dozens of copies of my books to government agencies. It is rare to get a response and when I do get one, it is typically an acknowledgment that they received the book. It is a similar story at the universities.

People are now reporting curing Autism with electromagnetically shielding the child's bedroom. This is consistent with Autism being an electromagnetic disease and may indeed be easily preventable. The Autism rates have been closely following the rise in cell phone towers and cell phones in the USA over the past decade. Transmitting Smart/AMR/AMI utility meters should be expected to increase the Autism rates, as they create a high powered antenna park at the home that is constantly transmitting pulsed radiation for approximately one mile in residential areas. Pulsed radiation is the most biologically harmful form of radiation transmission.

Electromagnetic shielding is a common response to the problem of unnatural man-made electromagnetic interference. You need to be very careful with shielding, as you can make the problem worse. I have been growing plants in Faraday cages and I have seen extensive growth problems occurring. Some people are inadvertently living in electromagnetically shielded homes and this may occur through the use of metal roofs, metal siding, foil radiant barriers, and insulation and windows that have electromagnetic shielding properties. Long term sickness may occur when living in such a home that may be accompanied by childhood development problems. You should not electromagnetically shield homes and workplaces as you may create radiation deficiency conditions in the inhabitants.

It is one of the dilemmas with RWS and EHS, to get sick from living in an unnaturally high man-made radiation environment, or to get sick from an electromagnetically screened natural radiation deficient environment. Either way, many humans will eventually get sick! Even pregnant mothers are electromagnetically shielding their unborn babies with a product called "Belly Armor". This action may eventually make them sick from radiation deficiency problems, similar to what astronauts show that live on the International Space Station for many months. The only known effective solution to RWS and EHS is to return your radiation environment back to natural levels.

Faraday cages are unnatural environments for humans and you should avoid living in one. My research into growing Dieffenbachia plants in Faraday cages is showing that they can show extensive stress inside them and may actually eventually die. A Faraday cage plant is shown in the next picture.

Electromagnetic shielding has problems as well and I have noticed that plants that come into contact with metal shielding may show stress and die back from the biologically harmful exposures. This is shown in the following picture.

Faraday Cage Biological Harm

This Dieffenbachia has spent eleven months living inside an ungrounded Faraday cage. It is showing extensive growth problems that include very small leaves, loss of patterning and abnormal branching structure.

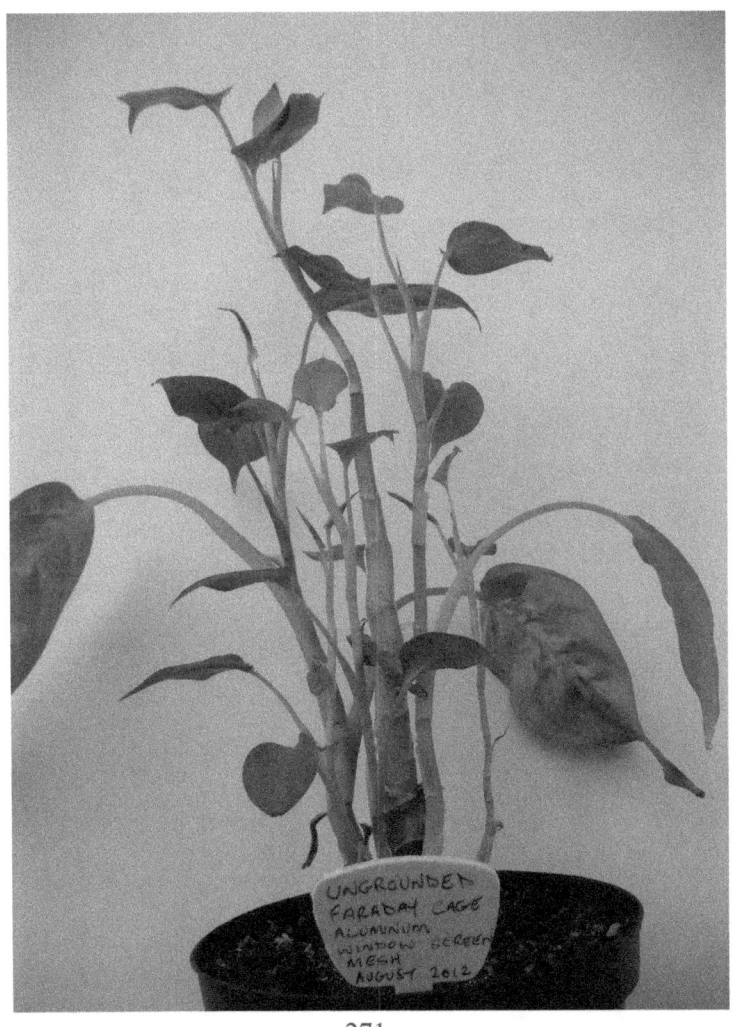

Electromagnetic Shielding Biological Harm

This Pyracantha bush came into contact with the aluminum mesh electromagnetic shield at the top of the wall and the plant died back from the biologically harmful exposure.

The human environment is no longer natural and this increasing of the man-made radiation environment should be expected to rapidly accelerate human evolution into an electromagnetically hardened animal. Unfortunately, many humans will die after many years of easily preventable illness and disease during this period that we are currently in.

The precursor to illness and disease are strange health conditions showing up. Radio Wave Sickness is well categorized today and the top reported radio wave sickness symptoms in order of frequency are:

1. *Fatigue.*

2. *Sleep disturbance.*

3. *Headaches.*

4. *Feeling of discomfort.*

5. *Difficulty in concentrating.*

6. *Depression.*

7. *Memory loss.*

8. *Visual disruptions.*

9. *Irritability.*

10. *Hearing disruptions.*

11. *Skin problems.*

12. *Cardiovascular.*

13. *Dizziness.*

14. *Loss of appetite.*

15. *Movement difficulties*

16. *Nausea.*

Source: Symptoms experienced by people in the vicinity of a cellular phone base station, Santini 2001, La Presse Medical.

Indeed, it is well known today that the sickness rates increase within approximately a quarter of a mile of a cell phone tower. The closer you are to it, the more likely it is for you to be sick. The utilities installing Smart/AMR/AMI meters at your home and in your neighborhood is comparable to turning your home into an antenna park.

When looking back in history we can find documented illnesses that are comparable to RWS and EHS:

- 1829 - Neurasthenia (Also called Americanitis or Nervosism): As a psychopathological term, Neurasthenia was used by George Miller Beard in 1869 to denote a condition with symptoms of fatigue, anxiety, excitation, restlessness, headache, neuralgia, pessimism, disturbed sleep and depressed mood. This condition showed up in the population during the construction of the railroads and the telegraph that shorted out the semiconductor properties of the natural ground and created electromagnetic interference. It was associated with upper class people and with professionals working in sedentary occupations.

- Mid 1800's - Female Hysteria: Women considered to be suffering from it exhibited a wide array of symptoms including faintness, nervousness, sexual desire, insomnia, fluid retention, heaviness in abdomen, muscle spasm, shortness of breath, irritability, loss of appetite for food or sex, and "a tendency to cause trouble". The women at the time were wearing steel hoop skirts and steel crinolines that would have been acting as antenna systems and Faraday cages to wireless energy.

- Early 1900's - Shenjing Shuairuo: Chinese equivalent of Neurasthenia. The condition is associated with a collection of symptoms including amnesia, dizziness, fatigue, gastrointestinal disorders, headaches, pain in joints and muscles, poor concentration and sexual dysfunction. This appears to match with the adoption of electricity into the cities.

In 1932, the German doctor Erwin Schliephake appears to be the first person to document the condition of Radio Wave Sickness. He noticed that the onset of symptoms were dependent upon the frequency and one particular frequency would bring on symptoms immediately, while a different frequency would take many hours of exposure to bring on the same conditions in a person. The onset followed this progression:

1. Initial reaction was extensive fatigue that would lead to apathy.

2. Long exposures would bring on classic Neurasthenia symptoms.

3. Prolonged exposure created a dull pressure in the head, headaches that would become intolerable, depression, inferiority, complaining, arguing, and uncertainty in dealing with others.

Dr. Erwin Schliephake found that the symptoms would resolve shortly after removal of the radio transmitter. In general, he found that low powered radio frequency (RF) would cause tranquilizing effects and high powered RF created irritation. The sensitivity was person dependent.

If you are currently experiencing the symptoms of RWS and EHS, I would recommend that you work on changing the electrical characteristics of your body. Changing the electrical characteristics of the human body can help to alleviate the symptoms of RWS and EHS. There are several proven ways to do this:

- **Change your fluid intake.**
- **Change your diet.**
- **Consume metal and electrolyte supplements.**

- **Exercise.**

- **Sweat.**

- **Go into a hot or cold environment.**

- **Build up muscle mass in every part of the body.**

- **Reduce or increase your weight.**

- **Submerge the body in water, such as a bath or swimming pool.**

- **Have no metal near to or in contact with the body.**

- **Have no electrical nor electronic products near to or in contact with the body.**

- **Wear a battery powered analogue watch with a second hand that has a non-conductive wrist strap.**

- **Wear clothes made out of natural materials.**

- **Make sure that you are not wearing shoes that create static.**

- **Wear conductive shoes or walk barefoot in areas that have no stray voltage problems nor excessive wireless radiation exposures.**

- **Sleep on the ground on a thin insulated mat to couple into it through capacitance. Make sure that there are no electrical cables in the ground.**

- **Sleep directly in contact with the ground in areas that do not have stray voltage problems.**

- **Remove metal from the body, such as dental fillings, dental implants and dental bridges.**

Regarding removing implants from the body, you should regard this as a last resort. There are many steps that you can take that may alleviate your symptoms and they are far easier than having implants removed. While metal implants are known for their ability to induce RWS and EHS into the human, you may be able to clear up the conditions without having to remove

276

these. Of course, if you do not have metal implants, then you should ensure that you do not get them in the future. They appear to interfere with the DC system of the body and act as antennas to wireless radiation.

A battery powered watch was a surprise to me. I had embedded a waterproof battery powered analogue watch with a resin strap and a second hand into the roots of a Dieffenbachia plant. The plant went on to display some of the best growth patterns that I have seen at my home. My home is filled with biologically toxic radio frequency emissions from transmitting utility meters and distant cell phone towers and my control plants typically show extensive deformity and retardation. The pulsing appears to mimic what happens when we walk barefoot in nature. Each step creates a pulse in the surrounding ground that the plants appear to respond favorably to. It appears I inadvertently made a discovery of profound importance.

You should be wary of watches with metal straps and digital watches as the effect is likely to be quite different with some of these models.

The analogue watch plant is shown in the next picture.

Using a Watch to Grow a Dieffenbachia Plant

The Dieffenbachia plant has a battery powered analogue watch with a resin strap and a second hand embedded in its roots. It is displaying growth patterns that far exceed that of my controls. It appears that the electromagnetic pulses that the watch emits creates radiation resistance in the plant. The watch used was a Casio men's MW600F-2AV 10-year battery sport watch.

You should pay attention to your pets. Looks for signs of RWS and EHS in them, as they can be an early warning sign that your environmental conditions are unnatural. I remember my grandfathers male dog always being sexually excited and aggressive. It would occasionally go crazy and run at full speed around the home for no reason. I suspect that he was walking the dog in areas that had stray voltage, stray currents and stray frequencies in them. My grandfather went on to die of Dementia which is associated with stray voltage, stray current and stray frequency exposure. He was probably being exposed to the same energies as the dog through the conductive dog leash and his leather soled shoes.

I have every expectation that in time, Dr. John Nash Ott will be recognized as the man who could have prevented the Autism epidemic and many other conditions as well! Dr. John Nash Ott was working in areas of "Inconvenient Truths" and the people who he was trying to inform about his valuable work simply ignored him, as it would have greatly affected their business model to acknowledge his work. Simply profits before people.

The modern human is derelict in its duty to the next generation who cannot protect themselves from harm. This madness must be stopped. The modern human is displaying apathy in the above areas that is leading to great levels of easily preventable sickness occurring in the current adult generations and retardation appearing in large numbers in the next generation. Indeed, experts in the field of Autism are indicating that at the currently accelerating levels, in fifteen years every USA child will have an Autism diagnosis!

"Radio Wave Sickness and Electromagnetic Hypersensitivity are easily preventable and one can only wonder how much longer the insanity of modern governments is going to be allowed to continue in this area."

Steven Magee

Radiation Resistance Process

The radiation resistance process is what much of the book has been talking about. Most people who live in modern cities are being bombarded by man-made electromagnetic radiation that has never existed in the history of the Earth. As such, you have no genetic adaptation nor natural protection to these new forms of environmental radiation exposures. Given that you cannot eliminate many of the radiation exposures that you are receiving, that puts you in the situation of building radiation resistance into the human mind and body to protect yourself from biological harm. This is the radiation resistance process that I am currently using:

- Eat fresh organic fruits and vegetables.

- Drink a pot of hot tea daily.

- Take a digestive supplement.

- Take an iodine supplement.

- Take a fish oil supplement.

- Wear a battery powered resin strap analogue wristwatch with a second hand to create DC pulses on the human body.

- Exercise daily to build muscle mass.

- Create a DC voltage on the human by supplementing with electrolytes and metals.

- Walk barefoot in rural areas where the ground is not electrified with stray voltage and the wireless radiation fields are low.

- Get your correct daily outdoor sunlight exposure in the shade of trees.

- Use rotational sleeping.

- Avoid spending extended time above 4,900 feet.

- Hibernate annually during winter.

The radiation resistance process will provide protection from radiation exposures, but will not guarantee that you may not develop sickness and possibly disease. These are preventative health steps that increase your chances of a long and healthy life.

People who have been excessively exposed to radiation typically do develop cancer many years or even decades later. Certain radiation exposures will probably eventually lead to cancer no matter what you do. However, it is proven that correct diet can delay progression of radiation exposures into disease. It is the reason why NASA uses organic vegetable and fruit based nutritional supplements on the International Space Station (ISS).

Radiation exposures do interfere with the digestive system and you should work with your doctor to identify supplements that can offset the radiation interference in the gut. I have found brewers yeast and a fiber supplement taken with each meal to be effective with aiding digestion in high radio wave fields. It is quite possible that the radio frequency environment is contributing to the new wave of super bugs that are being seen in the modern human.

Iodine is found in kelp and this offers a good natural source of it to protect your thyroid. Take the fish oil that matches your genetics, as your ancestors will have adapted to those sources of fish. Fish oil is known for its protective properties to the brain. NASA uses iodine and fish oil supplements on the ISS.

Many vitamin supplements are branded "energy" and people with Electromagnetic Hypersensitivity report that these do not work as advertised. Unfortunately, to completely clear up Electromagnetic Hypersensitivity you typically have to move out of the electromagnetic interference fields that are causing it. Currently, most people end up living on large house plots of multiple acres in rural forested areas and typically obtain great health in such locations.

The radiation resistance process takes time to work and you should use the techniques for at least one year before coming to any conclusions about them. You should be under the supervision and guidance of a qualified and licensed doctor who should tailor it for your particular needs.

"I keep dreaming of a future, a future with a long and healthy life, not lived in the shadow of cancer but in the light."

Patrick Swayze

Babies & Children

Raising babies and children has become a challenge for parents who want to have healthy offspring. We are living in a hazardous society that is marked by a corporate campaign of lie, confuse and deny in many areas that they are operating in. The corporate governments are suppressing corporate information that you are entitled to know through the simple action of silence. While it is unlikely that you will ever meet or be killed by a "terrorist", the probability that corrupt corporate and government activity will adversely impact your health and damage the development of your children is very high today.

As such, it is important that you protect your family and yourself. The people most at risk from damage are the babies. Young and rapidly dividing cells are very vulnerable. Their very thin skulls with the hole in the top puts babies brains at very high risk of damage from electromagnetic interference exposures. All testing for cell phones is done on a model of a very large adult human head, not a small baby's head. The least risk model was chosen as the cell phone testing standard, not the most risk model of the baby. You should be aware that having your cellphone near to your baby is a risky activity, as it was never tested in that dynamic.

All wireless products should be cleared from the home before bringing a baby into it. Have only the wireless products that you cannot do without and keep them far away from the baby. Be aware that the utility meters for the home commonly have high powered wireless transmitters in them and your baby should be raised in the bedroom that is furthest away from the radio frequency transmitting utility equipment. If you live near to high powered transmitters, then have the bedrooms tested and raise the baby in the lowest radio frequency contaminated bedroom.

The best place for the baby's cot is the center of the room. Walls typically have electrical cables and water pipes within them and both can emit electromagnetic fields that can extend several feet out from the wall. When placing the baby's cot in the center of the room, ensure that there are no electromagnetic fields from below that may affect the baby, such as an energy star electronic light, cable, or smoke detector mounted to the ceiling underneath if on an upper story. If you can, turn off the power in the baby's room to reduce field exposures. It is also prudent for the health of the entire family to turn off the electrical fuse board when you go to sleep and turn it back on when you wake up.

Toys are a problem and it is best to keep to basic traditional toys. Stay away from electrical, electronic and wireless toys. Lots of paper books and wooden building blocks are the way to go.

You should consider employing a building biologist before bringing a baby into the home. Building biologists are aware of the common home hazards that are easily avoidable. You would be surprised at how many health hazards are in your home that you simply are not aware of through lack of education.

You should remember that your baby has the genetics of an outdoor forest animal and that is where they are supposed to be raised. Ensure that during the daytime they get significant outdoor time around trees. When indoors, you should treat your baby as you would a shade houseplant. Keep them in bright rooms near to the window, but not in direct sunlight. Fresh air is important and either an open window or an air vent to the outdoors can help with this. Wikipedia states *In Japan, a forest bathing trip, called Shinrin-yoku in Japanese, Sanlimyok in Korean, is a short, leisurely visit to a forest and is regarded as being similar to natural aromatherapy.*

As your baby develops into a young child, you will likely get pressure for the latest electrical, electronic and wireless gadgets. Resist the pressure and limit TV and computer time. No TV or computer time is the best, but you are likely to have to assign a couple of hours per day limit for these activities. Unfortunately, most children are required to use computers in the corporate eduction system that we have. This is a very flawed policy considering what we know today about the negative health effects of electromagnetic interference exposures. Children really should be kept away from such exposures until they are fully developed into adults.

As your children develop, check for signs of fatigue, aggression, apathy, insomnia, or headaches. These are all signs of electromagnetic interference exposures. You should identify and remove such exposures to remedy these problems. If you have metal siding or foil radiant barrier home insulation, you should keep their beds and chairs away from the outer metal walls, as it may be absorbing and emitting energy, as well as electromagnetically shielding them from the natural Schumann resonances that are essential to good human health.

Make sure that they are not wearing static generating clothes or shoes. Identify and discard such items.

"It is easier to build strong children than to repair broken men."

Frederick Douglass

My Experiences

I started to play around with electricity when I was thirteen years old. Around that time I got my first home computer system which was to spark an interest in electricity and electronics. I left school at sixteen and became an apprentice electrician at the city center university research and teaching hospital. I worked in the electrical group for ten years and I have to say that I noticed people changing during that time.

I had noticed that some of the electricians had made the electrical rooms into workshops and they spent most of their day in them. In particular, there were two electricians who used to take their breaks in these rooms and sleep against the switchgear. They had very strange personalities!

In 1987 the hospital was in the process of switching over from conventional florescent lighting to electronic florescent lighting and installing computer systems for the medical records. There were robots in the sterile areas, ultrasonic baths, high frequency induction furnaces in the laboratories, RADAR operated automatic doors, and so on. I was working with many modern devices and no one ever warned me about the toxicity of these. In fact, no one ever told me about effects such as stray voltage, electromagnetic radiation health effects, harmonic energy making electromagnetic fields on cables get very large, pulsating magnetic fields affecting the brain, electrical and electronic field emissions and to stay out of them.

I would regularly walk through the hospital underground distribution system corridors and be inches from 6,600 volt AC electricity power cables and florescent lights. We would smash up the numerous florescent tubes that we would change every week, releasing toxic clouds of mercury contaminated white phosphor dust. Today, I can only imagine what these things must have been doing to my biological health!

The thing about working in a hospital is that you get to meet a lot of people who are sick and dying. I would have

many conversations with these people over the years. The consistent thing that they would repeatedly say to me is that they could not understand how they had become ill. It was always a mystery to them.

It is interesting that in 1987 Dr. John Nash Ott had actually published all of his research into electromagnetic radiation:

- My Ivory Cellar; [The Story of Time-Lapse Photography]. 1958.

- Health and Light: The Extraordinary Study That Shows How Light Affects Your Health and Emotional Well Being. 1973.

- Exploring the Spectrum: The Effects of Natural and Artificial Light on Living Organisms. 1975.

- Light, Radiation, and You: How to Stay Healthy. 1982.

- Color and Light: Their Effects on Plants, Animals and People. 1987.

Dr. John Nash Ott had discovered by 1987 that glass, artificial light sources, electricity, and electronic systems were having extensive detrimental effects on plants, animals, and humans. No one at the hospital was talking about it. The hospital had 1,000 beds, an animal research facility, a university research facility, a nursing teaching center, a doctors teaching center, a dental teaching center, and on site residence buildings to house all of the students. It was a huge university campus! One can only wonder why no one was talking about the toxicity of light, electricity, electronic systems and wireless radiation.

As well as my day job, I would go to college and university one day and one night per week. I obtained an Ordinary National Certificate, Higher National Certificate, Higher National Diploma, and a Bachelors with Honors in Electrical and Electronic Engineering. I can tell you that in ten years of studying electricity and electronics, not one mention was ever made of the toxicity of electricity.

Dr. John Nash Ott authored his last publication in 1987. I graduated in 1996, some nine years later. His work was never mentioned in any of my classes or text books on the subject. No teachings were given to me about the toxicity of electricity. Harmonics was taught, but only for its effects on electrical equipment, not human health. No mention was ever made about the very large electromagnetic fields that it puts onto cables and equipment.

One of the things that I remember as an apprentice was that when I started at the hospital, I was extremely fatigued for the first few months of working there. The mechanical apprentice who started at the same time as me was reporting the same thing. Today, I know that effect to be the body adjusting to toxic environmental conditions.

Both the mechanical apprentice and myself were from rural areas outside of the city. Working at a highly industrialized facility in the city center was an alien environment for us. In addition to the variety of modern equipment that the hospital had, it had a large number of telecommunications radio frequency transmission antenna systems on the roof. Today it is known that these systems are harmful to the human at close proximity. We were constantly working near the antenna systems with no precautions.

I had found the people in the facilities team to be mostly pleasant, but a little strange too. I had also noticed personalities changing during the ten years that I worked in this group, my own personality was also changing. In particular, I do remember one of the members of the electrical team being exceptionally friendly and very smart and he actually became the opposite, unfriendly and mean during the time I knew him. The adoption of electronics and computer systems into the hospital had become rampant during that time period. This particular person had a number of metal implants that today we know to be incompatible with exposure to the various forms of electricity.

I had noticed that my face was constantly flushing and that my memory was having issues. Forgetfulness was quite normal during my time there and I was always tired. My mating cycle was frequently being triggered and I thought it was normal. I had never known any different.

In 1996 I changed my position and started working with dialysis machines. These were highly complex computer controlled machines that were filled with the latest electrical and electronic products. The joke in the group was that everyone who joined the team got divorced shortly afterwords! Little did they know that it was the electromagnetic radiation emissions from the machines that was probably causing it.

I had noticed my health significantly degrading in my late twenties after joining this group. General aches and pains, feeling lethargic, nosebleeds, gums bleeding after brushing my teeth and being extremely tired in the mornings had become normal. Getting up in the mornings was always difficult. Working on my home during the weekends was a problem due to the low energy levels. I later realized that part of this may have been coming from drinking reverse osmosis water. The dialysis team was making its tea and coffee with the same reverse osmosis water that the machines used! Reverse osmosis water is highly processed water that is extremely mineral deficient!

It was the first position that had issued me with a laptop computer system, anti-static strap, and pager. I remember seeing the doctor about recurring chapped lips that had shown up in this position and they told me it was normal. I now know that it was exposure to the artificial light from the laptop computer that was causing this. The pager was constantly clipped to my belt and would work throughout the region, so I know that I was in extensive unnatural radio fields that communicated with it. I would have the pager with me, even when I slept. I do wonder if the early pager systems had harmful biological emissions from them? I was also being exposed to stray voltage and stray frequencies from the anti-static strap which is extensively documented in the diary industry for making farmers, their families, and their animals sick.

The first person that I knew who committed suicide was in this group. I will always be curious to know if it was caused in part from the toxic exposures that he received during his time in it. He was in the group for many years, as opposed to the three years that I worked there.

In 1999 I went to live in La Palma in the Canary Islands and started to work at an altitude of approximately 7,755 feet. I was working with telescope drive systems that were controlled by industrial computer systems. There are no doubts that sunlight in the right dose is an excellent medication! Living in the Canary Islands did wonders for improving my health. However, it was short lived.

I noticed that the longer I was in the position in the Canary Islands, the sicker I was getting. Like many people in this situation, I did not understand what was happening. Today, I do believe that I was actually sitting in the fields of the neighbors cathode ray tube (CRT) television when I was at home. The problem with CRT televisions is that they have extensive fields around them and those fields will pass straight through walls! Their television was on the other side of the wall from my sofa.

I had also been issued with a laptop computer at work and I was constantly working on it. Email had become a popular form of communication. There were no warnings given about laptop computers and human health. I now know that many laptop computers have unnatural magnetic fields around them, emit electromagnetic interference, and that their displays can induce health problems into the human.

I purchased my first cellphone in La Palma. I had noticed after having it for a while that it would cause strange noises on my stereo system in the car. I now understand this to be the cellphone logging into the cellphone tower every ten minutes or so. The transmission was so powerful from the cellphone that it was interfering with the stereo system!

I lived in two properties in La Palma and the second property was a home that was in the countryside. I only lived in that home for a short period before leaving for my next position in Hawaii. However, I had noticed that my girlfriend was constantly complaining of headaches there and my health was continuing to decline. Today, I suspect that it was the street lights that were outside of the home. Many street lights create a toxic form of light to the human, create stray voltage, and they can have strange electromagnetic emissions from them.

I moved to the USA in 2001 and lived in Waimea on the island of Hawaii. I was walking to and from work under the high voltage power lines that ran through the streets there. During that time I had noticed that I was getting very anxious and that if I was placed in a stressful situation that my heartbeat would start to race and my face would flush. Today I attribute that health effect to the high voltage power lines, as it cleared up when I moved away from Waimea.

Working at 13,796 feet is well known to be harmful to human health and most people on the mountain were in some state of sickness. We were commuting up and down the mountain daily and our bodies were constantly in a state of confusion. I knew from conversations with other staff members that poor health was a feature of daily high altitude commuting. Pilots, air hostesses, and frequent fliers suffer from the same thing.

At 13,796 feet very little grows! It is a barren landscape that is just rocks and cinder. When you work at altitude you notice that trees stop growing at a very definite altitude. This line of demarcation is called the "Tree Line". It appears to be an effect of radiation exposure. As you increase in altitude, the air gets thinner and less solar radiation filtering is taking place. More energy is in the electromagnetic spectrum and it appears to move outside of what the trees can survive in. You will find very strange growth patterns in the trees near the tree line with unusual branching and weird deformities. For this reason, I advise people to be very careful with high altitude radiation exposure. If there are no trees around at altitude, then you should avoid the sunlight, as it may give you a very strange type of radiation sickness!

In 2003, I joined the astronomy team and moved onto the night shift. I had suspected that living on the mountain for a week and having a week off would be healthier and it was! I also started to build a solar photovoltaic powered home in Hawaii. Everything was going well, until I moved into the home. The home was powered by a modified sine wave inverter that was ran off high capacity 24 volt batteries that were charged by 8 solar photovoltaic modules. Like most off-grid homes, it had "Energy Star" compact florescent lighting (CFL) throughout the home.

I had noticed that there was a constant buzzing on the phone line whenever I would use it. I spoke with the electrician who had installed it and I was advised that it was a feature of off-grid homes. I was developing a wide variety of health issues the longer that I lived in the home. The main health symptom was fatigue. The longer I lived there, the more excessive the fatigue got. I got to the point where I would drink energy drinks and then go to bed and sleep. The drinks were having no effect on me! However, my mating cycle was constantly being triggered.

Today, I realize that the buzzing on the phone line was a combination of dirty electricity on the electrical grounding system combined with radio wave emissions from the electrical wiring. The effect was made worse during the night from the compact florescent lights (CFL) putting harmonics onto the cables and the electromagnetic fields that they emit. I did not know it at the time, but I had developed Radio Wave Sickness (RWS)!

I knew two other people who lived in off-grid solar powered homes very well. One was extremely passive aggressive with most people and his personality was lacking empathy. The other was showing severe symptoms of forgetfulness. When you explore the field of dirty electricity, you find that the off-grid homes generally have the poorest power quality. The quality of electricity will vary with the loads on the system. It is likely that this dirty electricity was a source of their problems.

I developed intestinal pains during working on the night shift and about every two weeks I would get painful

cramps that would lead to diarrhea. I did not know it at the time, but it is classical symptoms of shifting solar radiation exposure. It would generally occur on my first day off in sunlight after working a week of nights.

The second person that I knew who committed suicide had worked at this facility. He was a welder. Welders get exposed to significant levels of stray voltage, stray currents, stray frequencies, ultraviolet light and various electromagnetic radiation emissions from their arc welding equipment. Both of the people I have worked with who committed suicide were nice people. Unfortunately, it is well known that electromagnetic radiation exposures can make nice people do strange things that are out of character for them.

In 2006 I changed jobs and went to work in Tucson, Arizona. This signified a move back onto normal utility electricity. The strange thing was, I had noticed the same effect occurring that I had noticed when I started working in the hospital. I was constantly fatigued in this position to the point of almost falling asleep every day in the first few months.

I was spending four hours per day in transportation systems and eight hours at the observatory. The interesting thing is, I had measured the voltage waveform on the electrical system there and it was highly distorted. This distortion creates large amounts of harmonic energy on the electrical system and puts very large fields on the wiring and equipment. I did not realize the implications of that at the time, because I had never been taught that electromagnetic radiation emissions and electrical system harmonics were harmful!

I remember when I saw it that I was surprised. Out at the telescope it was a highly distorted voltage sine wave. However, at the uninterruptible power supply (UPS), it was an almost perfect voltage sine wave. The sine wave got better the closer to the UPS system and worse the further away from it. I suspect that electronically generated sine waves do not travel well over distances, particularly when they are feeding into electronic products. It is likely that the different frequencies of energy in electronically generated AC voltage sine waves start to interact with cables and the electronic products that they supply and this may distort them.

I later hired a contractor to assist with work at the observatory and it was not long before I was hearing the same story from him, he was getting really fatigued too! Today, I attribute the fatigue problems to the electromagnetic fields that were created by the harmonic energy on the electrical system.

At home, my relationship was problematic and within a year we had broken up. All I wanted to do was lay in bed, as my energy levels were so low. I could not sleep much, as I had insomnia constantly. I was getting intestinal pains and diarrhea a few times every month. I had to stop exercising in 2007 as I would get chest pains and breathing difficulties!

During my time in this position I had developed very strange facial and head pains. They would come and go and I had no idea what it was. I started to go to the doctor and was sent for many tests. No one could tell me what it was. During researching the book "Toxic Electricity", I realized that my seat at the office was next door to the telescope electrical room that contained all of the control systems, WiFi router, networks, and computers! I was sitting next to a laser printer and nearby was the cordless phone. I had been sitting in very large electromagnetic fields every day. The fact that my company wireless laptop computer also had large electromagnetic emissions coming out of it did not help.

The longer that I was in the position, the more aches and pains I was getting. My skin was getting to be so hot and painful that I was having daily baths to try and calm it down. The funny thing was, I looked perfectly normal on the outside! No one would have been aware that my health was failing. Insomnia was a big issue and it was rare that I would get a good nights sleep.

Anxiety became a significant problem and it was getting worse with time. I knew I was being poisoned, I just could not figure out the source of the poison!

I later reported that I had identified a number of environmental health issues to the management team of this facility in 2012, after I had published the book "Toxic Electricity". I did not tell them what I had identified, as I was interested to see if they would want to know. Unfortunately, their response to the problems was silence. Responding with silence to inconvenient truths is a common problem in the workplace today and is a major problem with the prevalence of Sick Building Syndrome (SBS). Many managers know that their facilities are causing their staff to be sick, but simply stay silent about it. What I found most concerning about this is that it was an Ivy League college and university that specializes in human health!

I joined the solar industry in 2008 and by this time fatigue, insomnia, occasional intestinal pains and diarrhea, hot skin, and general aches and pains throughout my body had become something that I had accepted as aging. My doctor was informing me that it was a normal aspect of aging, everyone is the same! Staying awake on the job was getting to be a significant problem.

I eventually started to see the doctor for medication to keep me awake in order to keep working. I was taking a medication called "Provigil". It keeps you awake for exactly sixteen hours from the point of taking it. The military issue it to the troops during wars to prevent the troops from sleeping when they are under attack. It is an amazing medication and worked well for me. However, it does not make the original problems go away, it simply masks them. It also costs approximately $400 per month!

Needless to say, I was not looking for a tablet, I was looking for a cure!

I had developed red blotchy patches of skin on my buttocks. They were not painful nor sore. I had noticed them in the mirror after showering one day. They were there for months. I saw the doctor about them and they did not know what would cause it. Today, I suspect that it was the company cellphone electromagnetic emissions that were causing them, as I would keep the mobile phone in my back pocket. They cleared up after I left that company and I have never seen them since. The blotchy skin effect is reported by people who have Electromagnetic Hypersensitivity.

During my development of the book "Toxic Electricity", I analyzed the environment that I was working in. I was working in a cubicle desk that was surrounded by other workers who had cellphones and wireless computer systems. My desk was very close to the electrical room that housed all of the computer network equipment for the building and the wireless router. The high voltage overhead utility power lines and poles in the street were approximately 30 feet from my desk! The airport was across the road and there would have been extensive RADAR and radio wave emissions from it. There may have been infra-sound and pollution issues as well. The company used radio frequency identification (RFID) controlled doors and I would pass through these perhaps 100 times per day to get between departments. I was also sitting near to the transmitting RFID door sensor, carrying a company smart phone and my own personal cell phone.

In 2009 I commissioned a very large utility solar power system over two months. It was an interesting experience that was setting the stage for finding the cure that I was looking for.

During the two months of commissioning, I had noticed some very strange behaviors in the people involved with the project. I was seeing aggressiveness, fatigue, and forgetfulness. I was also seeing habitual lying over commissioning issues that were showing up and that appeared to be caused by pressure for the project to be perceived as successful by the company management team. In conversations with the staff, they were telling me that they were not sleeping well and that they were having aches and pains throughout their bodies. Very similar conditions to my own!

One day, after spending the entire day working around the high voltage transformers, electronic power inverter systems, and solar modules, I noticed that my smell was off. At the time, I was in the 24,000 volt switching center at the site and I could smell smoke when there was no smoke. The most amount of electrical power was in here, as it feeds into the electrical utility transmission system. It was a sunny day with approximately eighteen million watts of electronically generated harmonic electricity flowing through the room. There was approximately 10% harmonic distortion on the utility power sine wave.

I was absolutely convinced that something was on fire and the people that I was with were telling me that they could not smell it. I also appeared to be intoxicated. Later that day, I found that I could not stop drinking due to an insatiable thirst! I had been drinking during the day and I did not appear to be dehydrated, my urine wasn't dark, nor was I sunburned as I had sunscreen on, sunglasses, a wide brimmed hard hat, and a whole body arc flash suit. Everything appeared to be back to normal the next day.

During research for my books, I found that these symptoms are listed as Radio Wave Sickness (RWS). I was not surprised, as the power plant was producing excessive harmonics and nobody had warned me about the dangers of high powered electronic utility equipment that has excessive harmonic energy on it.

After leaving this project, I soon discovered that I could not remember computer passwords, phone numbers, alarm codes, and basic mathematics was difficult for me. It was clear that I had received a toxic brain exposure from the high powered electronic utility equipment. Nikola Tesla documents having a similar experience during his research and development.

I started to develop books on solar power systems and that led to the discovery of the multiple-Sun effect. The multiple-Sun effect occurs anywhere that there are solar reflections taking place. Solar power systems with their reflective glass surfaces create it. I knew the effect was important and I started to develop it further. I found that it also occurs in city environments where there are large amounts of glass in buildings. It is particularly bad around glass covered tower buildings.

The multiple-Sun effect significantly raises the radiation levels in the human environment to above the radiation levels of Space. Bingo! I had discovered that I had

developed radiation sickness over the years of extended exposure to radiation sources.

I also stopped taking the medications. I had been taking Provigil for the daytime and over the counter sleeping tablets to counteract the insomnia symptoms. This over the counter sleep medication was a range of melatonin, diphenhydramine, and doxylamine succinate. The doctor has prescribed Seroquel, but I found that it made me feel really bad for the first hour in the morning.

The interesting thing is, it is commonly reported in the USA that approximately 50% of the population is taking prescription medications! I had noticed on my travels that many people that I have worked with are routinely taking medications. I was not alone in this lifestyle that had developed over the years. Unfortunately, many USA children are also in the same situation.

Within days I went into really severe drugs withdrawal. I literally could not get out of bed for a few days as I felt so bad. Flu like symptoms followed by really bad headaches for about two weeks that would not respond to medication. I had never experienced this before!

It slowly cleared up which led me to the understanding that if you take medications long term, then your mind and body will go toxic. The interesting thing was, my thought patterns changed! A calm mind replaced a mind that was constantly active with various thoughts. My insomnia also slowly cleared up. As such, it is better to avoid the medications if you can.

After doing the work with the development of the multiple-Sun effect in 2010, I knew that it was wise to balance it out and to spend a corresponding amount of time out of the Sun. For six months, I avoided sunlight. A few weeks into this process, I got extremely ill with flu like symptoms. My heartbeat was fluctuating and I had intense pains throughout my body. It was so bad that I thought that I was going to die! It lasted a few days and then slowly got better. It was clear at this point that I was in radiation withdrawal. About a month into the withdrawal I had my blood tested and everything was showing normal levels.

Extreme fatigue followed for a few months and that eventually cleared up. I noticed that several weeks into the withdrawal process that my body was reacting to sunlight exposure, if I spent time outside in the sunlight, then I would have a big headache the next day.

I went to view Niagara falls with my friends and we rode right up to the bright white wall of water on the Maid of the Mist. For me, it was like drinking several beers, it made me develop symptoms of intoxication!

As time went by, my pains started to subside. Eventually, they disappeared! Today, after years of random aches and pains, I am pain free.

After several months of avoiding the Sun, I had my blood tested again and it had gone low in both vitamin B12 and vitamin D. My diet had not changed, the only thing that had changed was my sunlight exposure. The vitamin D deficiency was expected, as it is well documented as being a photosynthesis vitamin. There was plenty of meat and fish in my diet for sources of B12, so being low on B12 was a surprise. So I concluded that the B12 deficiency was related to the lack of Sun exposure.

It is interesting to note that in Autistic children, vitamin B12 injections have been shown to significantly reduce their symptoms. I do currently believe that both Autism and Attention Deficit Disorder (ADD) are electromagnetic diseases.

I started to get 15 minutes of Sun per day, which is the current guidelines for maintaining adequate vitamin D levels. Much to my surprise, I eventually got to a period where extreme fatigue showed up and all that I wanted to do was sleep every day. My vitamin D and B12 levels appeared to continue to decline and had brought on the symptoms of Seasonal Affect Disorder (SAD). I increased the sunlight exposure time to an hour per day in the shade and that eventually fixed it.

Toxic Health © Steven Magee

Just for curiosity, I actually started to sunbathe and found that at two hours per day, the aches and pains came back. They were simply fixed by staying out of the Sun for a few days. I eventually established that my outdoor solar radiation levels are at 1 hour per day in the shade in sunny Arizona to maintain good health. My genetics are a mix of Irish and English with relatively white skin. My skin today is a golden brown. If you have darker skin, then your daily requirements for solar radiation exposure will be higher due to the pigmentation. I later realized that the aches and pains may have been caused by the high wireless radiation levels outside, as my plants were showing deformities in that area. Some parts of my garden have wireless radiation levels of approximately 700 millivolts per meter, which is considered very high by most electromagnetic radiation researchers. In the National Park forest, the wireless energy meter reads zero.

At this point, the main problem that I was showing was occasional fatigue. It was the kind of fatigue that makes you want to take a nap in the middle of the day. During research for the book "Toxic Electricity" I had realized that people who report Electromagnetic Hypersensitivity generally report fatigue. I started to research my human body voltage and found that there was a large AC waveform riding on my body. Turning off my home electrical circuits eliminated it. I also discovered that my tiled flooring in the home was electrified with "Stray Voltage" from the electrical utility neutral and started to wear slippers when home to prevent coming into contact with it. I changed all of my light bulbs from compact florescent lights (CFL) to conventional filament lights. I tested the CFL's and found that they had unnatural spectrums of light and radio wave emissions. I switched over to a diet rich in organic fresh fruit and vegetables and turned off the cell phone. These actions brought up my energy levels.

I should mention that due to my knowledge of how utility power companies willfully mislead the public, during the Fukushima nuclear disaster I changed my diet over to dried and canned food in March 2011 to avoid the surge of radiation contaminated food in the USA food system. During the following nine months, I noticed that my skin started to develop problems on my elbows with rough, dry, and brittle skin. My teeth started to decay, and I was getting indigestion and stomach problems. Heart burn and acid reflux was an issue and I was constantly taking antacids to alleviate the symptoms. These problems fixed themselves after a few months of eating fresh organic food.

I concluded that extended exposure to preserved food is harmful to human health and the health problems can be simply fixed by eating fresh organic food.

I had noticed that the occasional fatigue completely cleared up when I went camping in remote National Parks, which I would do at least once per year. To clear the occasional fatigue up, I suspected that I was going to have to move to a different area, due to the high radiation levels around my property from the three cell phone towers that are approximately between 2,000 feet to 2,300 feet from my home. I had planted trees and plants around my property when I purchased it and I knew that they would eventually reduce the radio frequency radiation levels by absorbing it.

Watching the plants grow over the years led me to the understanding that things were not growing correctly in the garden. The extensive indoor plant experiments that I was performing showed me that the electromagnetic radiation environment of the entire home was extremely unnatural, as even my control plants were deforming! I had many Dieffenbachia (Dumb Cane) plants in the home and every one was deformed! There were zones around the outside of the home that were showing stress and growth problems in the plants. These were the entire west side of the home and the entire north east side of the home where the utility electrical equipment was located. The northwest part of the garden was the worst and there were areas that I had noticed that the plants would die when placed there. It did not matter what type of plant I planted in these locations, they would die after several months.

I took all of my wireless devices out of service in summertime 2012 and had the electrical utility company

change out the automatic meter reader (AMR) for a conventional mechanical electric meter on both my home and the neighbors home. This appears to have cured some of the growth problems that I was seeing in my plants. It was clear that the utility company and my wireless devices had inadvertently turned my home and garden area into the equivalent of an antenna park! It improved the occasional fatigue, but did not fully clear it up. I did get very sore and sensitive teeth in the weeks following removing the wireless products, as did my neighbors. It appeared to be a withdrawal symptom from the wireless radiation. In summertime 2013 I had the first ever fruits that the garden had produced from a peach and a pomegranate tree. It was obvious that the wireless radiation exposures had been causing these trees to abort their fruit development in the previous years.**

Many people report problems with metal coil mattresses. I checked mine out and found that it was acting as an antenna system for AC electricity and radio waves! I changed out my metal coil mattress to a latex mattress to see if that would help. It improved my sleep, but did not appear to improve the occasional fatigue.

I tried the "Earthing" health technique for two reasons. I wanted to assess it for my book "Toxic Electricity" and I thought that it may clear up the fatigue. I saw my back tingle for about a week in the area where I was in contact with the earthing cable, so it definitely was doing something. However, as time went on I got the most severe bad back that I have ever had. It was in the base of my spine and badly affected my walking! It took a few weeks to clear up. Then I went into the worst period of heart arrhythmia that I have ever experienced! Fearing a heart attack, I decided to stop the technique. I tested the cable and found that it was acting as an antenna system and had a wide range of frequencies on it! The grounding cable health technique did not work for me, but there are people who say that it does work.

People had commented over the years that when they would enter my home that there was a strange odor. I had wondered for a long time where this odor was coming from,

as I had noticed it myself from time to time. It was apparent when coming into the home after it had been locked up for several hours. I found that my kitchen island had an in-line sewer vent valve installed into it. These valves allow air to enter into the sewer system from the home and prevent the sewer gas from escaping. When the in-line vent valve ages, it may start to leak sewer gas. Replacing this fixed the odor problem. If you have one of these valves in your home, you should pay attention to it as sewer gas is explosive and poisonous!

I followed Dr. John Nash Ott's advice and installed ultraviolet (UV) transmitting plastic in the areas of my home where I spend my daytime. When compared to the crystal clear UV transmitting acrylic windows, my double glazed glass windows look green and dim! This heavily filtered colored light from the low-E double glazed glass windows appears to have been contributing to the fatigue issues that I was seeing. Using "full spectrum" glazing appears to have significantly reduced the occasional fatigue problem.

The health benefits that I observed during the initial few weeks of testing ultraviolet transmitting acrylic windows were:

- Excellent daytime energy levels.

- Wonderful sleep cycle.

- Improved mental functioning.

- Brighter indoor environment.

- Indoor colors are vivid.

- The computer is more pleasant to work with. It appears to have significantly reduced the dry eyes and chapped lips that it gave me with long periods of use.

- Fruits ripen faster in the full spectrum light.

- Good health.

In the first month that I installed this I did see some interesting aches and pains. My left ankle and my right elbow were aching for no reason whatsoever. I then got some intestinal pains that I have not had before. They cleared up after a few weeks and appeared to be due to the changes that were taking place in my body.

After the initial surge in health, I started getting the desire to occasionally nap again at lunchtime. I have established that I get full health whenever I go camping in remote National Parks or travel to areas that are rural with very low cell phone reception. While I have always associated good health with low cell phone reception, I do spend more time outside around nature on these trips.

I increased my outdoor time to two hours around solar noon in the shade. Generally I will read a book during this time. I will get a little direct sunlight exposure also, typically half an hour. This really brought up my energy levels.

This leads me to conclude that exposure to the peak in solar radiation that occurs around solar noon is essential to good health. My daily solar radiation exposure is to sit near to my shady ultraviolet transmitting full spectrum acrylic window while I develop my research and then to go out around solar noon for a couple of hours in the shade reading. I'll take a stroll around the garden in the direct sunlight during that time.

I moved my computer next to the shady ultraviolet transmitting window. When I work on it during the daytime, I now have the outdoors in my field of view. This enables my eyes, face and hands to get full spectrum daylight exposure all day long. My daytime light environment is now in tune with thousands of years of evolution. One could say that I have finally achieved resonance with the daylight environment!

I also discovered that the gas company installed an automatic meter reader (AMR) radiation transmitting device at my property during this time. I do not know exactly when it was installed, but I asked around and it appears that it was installed sometime in January 2013. It was the reason why my health took a step back. The gas company installed them throughout the community, as I could see the same shiny AMR meters at other properties in the neighborhood. I tested it and it was emitting a radiation pulse every several seconds. The previous gas meter had no detectable radiation pulses coming from it. I am now watching my plants in that area to see if they are going to deform, go dormant, or die.

To reduce the toxic effects of this, I have now moved my desk as far away from the AMR gas meters that I can in the home. It is simply the prudent thing to do. The World Health Organization class wireless transmitting devices as "Possibly Carcinogenic". There are no shortage of people who have traced their health problems to these devices and one can only wonder why they have not been banned. Moving further away from the AMR transmitters increased my energy levels which tells me that they are affecting my health. The symptoms that I have observed are:

- January: Fatigue.
- February: Fatigue, waking up feeling hung over and lethargic.
- March: Fatigue, waking up feeling hung over and lethargic, fuzzy thinking and concentration problems.
- April: I abandoned my bed and started to sleep on the floor. I also increased the electromagnetic screening around the transmitting AMR meters. This reduced the severity of the symptoms.

I notified both the gas company and the Federal Communication Commission (FCC) that they were causing harmful biological interference at my property and to remove the AMR transmitting devices from the vicinity of my home.

In March 2013 I started to get really sick with classic Radio Wave Sickness symptoms. This is how the sickness progressed:

- Day 1 - Fuzzy thinking.
- Day 2 - Dizziness, fuzzy thinking, headaches.
- Day 3 - Dizziness, fuzzy thinking, headaches, insomnia.
- Day 4 & 5 - Dizziness, fuzzy thinking, headaches, insomnia, fatigue.

I had seen this range of symptoms appear with a similar rapid progression back in summertime 2012 when I went to stay in a mountaintop forest vacation area. When I researched the location from satellites I found that I had been staying just a few hundred meters from a large antenna park that had cell phone towers and multiple radome installations in it! The interesting thing was, my girlfriend showed a different rate of progression. She was symptom free until the fourth day when she started showing headaches, insomnia and fatigue. We were both relieved to leave that location and our symptoms rapidly subsided within hours of leaving the area.

It was clearly Radio Wave Sickness that had shown up, but what was causing it? My best guess was that I had moved into a hotspot of radiation and that it was affecting me. It was the correct assumption. I had been given a printer to repair and was using it daily to test it. I had noticed that it had built in WiFi but was not using it. I tested the printer with my radio frequency meter and there was a large field of wireless radiation around it! I had been sitting just 2 feet away from the printer in a 1,000 mV/m radiation field daily and this was consistent with the symptoms that had shown up. It appears that wireless network printers exhibit a similar behavior to wireless network routers and continually fill the area with microwave radiation. It is for this reason that you should not sit near to devices like this. The best way is simply not to have wireless devices of any kind.

I had noticed that the ultraviolet acrylic windows were reacting to infra-sound. A pulse of energy would hit them and make them vibrate. It is very noticeable at my home and lasts less than a second. There is no wind present when I have seen this occur. Out in the desert is a military bombing range that generates sonic booms. When I worked on Kitt Peak, I would hear the sonic booms frequently and they would shake the buildings! It appears that I am now detecting them at my home with my acrylic windows! This is concerning, as infra-sound is well known for its ability to make people sick.

In May 2013 I found that my toilets were electrified with stray voltage. When I would urinate into them this would make the drain wet and electrify them from the stray voltage in the street! I was curious and tested my showers and found that when the drain gets wet, it electrifies the shower! This is a concerning development, as it means that there are many toilets out there that are electrified with stray voltage. This is consistent with some trips that I took to the doctors several years ago with urethra problems that the doctor could not diagnose. I suspect that the stray voltage issue was much higher during that period. I only saw it for one year and then it spontaneously cleared up. Needless to say, now I know that my drains are electrified, I no longer urinate into my toilets. This action increased my energy levels. I did see quite severe headaches occur during the following two weeks that gradually subsided and this appeared to be a withdrawal reaction.

High activity muscle building exercise was a step that I had wanted to introduce for quite some time. I was reluctant to start doing it while I was dealing with and characterizing the earlier issues. I have always walked for exercise during this recovery process but I wanted to introduce a daily exercise regimen that made me really sweaty! Walking is not really exercise, as it does not work the entire body. This was evidenced by my weight increasing from 154 pounds in 2009 to 192 pounds in 2013. During that period I had led a sedentary life with most of my time spent at home. I started to follow a DVD workout routine every day. I lost 6 pounds in the first ten days!

The thing that was very noticeable was that my hunger subsided and that I was content with smaller portions. My body shape change was noticeable as was my increase in muscle mass. After twenty days my weight had stabilized at 184 pounds and it was obvious that my fat was in the process of being converted into muscle, as the exercise routine had become enjoyable and my strength had significantly increased. By thirty days my stamina had developed and I was able to fully perform each exercise routine.

While I was setting up a structured water plant experiment, it caused me to investigate what exactly was in my drinking water filter. I had been advised by numerous people in Tucson to filter my water, as they believed that the drinking water was contaminated by industrial and mining activities in the area. I thought that I was carbon filtering my water. However, when I checked the water filter box, I found that there were ion exchange resin beads in addition to carbon. It appears that since 2007 that I was drinking carbon filtered ion exchanged water! I checked the filters out on the internet and sure enough, I found many complaints about them from people who had been made ill by using them. Naturally, I switched my drinking water back to standard faucet water from the utility company. Over the following weeks I saw my energy levels increase.

The gas company did eventually remove the biologically harmful AMR meter from my home. However, they refused to remove the one on the neighbors home just 15 feet away! I had actually requested that they remove four of their transmitting meters from within 100 feet of my bedrooms, but only the one on my home was changed for a non-transmitting meter. The gas company knows that these transmitting meters make me sick, but are okay with that state of affairs. It is clearly a case of willful biological assault with known biologically harmful radio frequency devices that the military weaponized as they were so good at making the enemy sick! And it is happening at my home which represents my greatest financial investment! My home is not a place of safe refuge and this is a violation of the USA Declaration of Independence.

Heart arrhythmia and insomnia eventually showed up when I was sleeping on the floor. It was likely a combination of extended exposure to the transmitting utility meters in the area and the summertime stray voltage levels increasing on the concrete floor that I was sleeping on. This required a change in direction to seek good health.

The many plant experiments that I was performing with the Dieffenbachia plant had started to yield results that I had not expected. Some of the plants instead of extensively deforming were actually showing growth that was closer to the normal growth that the plants were displaying when I bought them. These experiments were:

- **Growing a Dieffenbachia with a battery powered analogue watch with a second hand embedded in its roots.**

- **Growing a Dieffenbachia by watering it with hot tea that had cooled.**

- **Growing a Dieffenbachia by connecting a single cell 1.5 volt battery connected between the roots and the leaves.**

- **Growing a Dieffenbachia by grounding the roots and soil to the conductive tiled floor. (Note: This only worked on the tiled floor furthest from the street and the utility electrical equipment.)**

So I started to wear the same model of resin strap battery powered analogue watch, drink tea, connect myself to a 1.5 volt battery between the sole of my foot and wrist, and walk barefoot on the tiled floor furthest from the street.

Connecting to the 1.5 volt single cell battery caused me to develop very strong chemical smelling urine that was a similar odor to WD-40. The strong smelling urine had me concerned, so I stopped connecting to a battery and decided to instead turn my body into a battery! It is easily achieved by ingesting electrolyte and metal supplements. A positive voltage of 0.5 volts at the finger relative to the grounded feet was developed using this process. This turned on the chemical smelling urine again. The urine chemical smell disappeared after a few months of taking the supplements and seemed to be a reaction to the 0.5 volts DC that had developed on the body.

I was seeing poor digestion over the years that was marked by loose stools. I had become aware at this point that the extensive radio frequency fields that were passing through my home were interfering with the digestive system. This can be remedied by taking a digestive supplement. The most effective supplement that I identified was brewers yeast. I started taking a teaspoon dissolved in a glass of water with every meal.

The occasional fatigue and high pitched "microwave hearing" buzzing ears are the only regular health symptoms that I display today, along with the damage to my memory that occurred in 2009 at the high powered solar photovoltaic utility power plant. The fatigue is mild and tends to occur around noon and disappears by the evening. I am wondering if it is following the solar radiation power levels, as I only see it appear when it peaks at solar noon. Solar noon appears to trigger the fatigue and sunset eliminates it. It is an interesting phenomenon that appears to be tied to the peak in daily radiation levels! Wireless radiation induced fatigue is documented in the book "Insomnia, Fatigue and Cell Phone Towers" by Conrad LeBeau. In 1932, the German doctor Erwin Schliephake appears to be the first person in history to document the condition of Radio Wave Sickness, with fatigue being the primary feature of the sickness.

I had been wondering how much of the occasional fatigue was coming from the electrical transmitting utility meters. I got my answer in 2013 when we had a daytime power cut for several hours. The longer the power cut went on for, the bigger my headache became! It was clearly a withdrawal headache from the changed radiation environment, as the electrical meters stop broadcasting radiation when the power is off. There are no doubts that the electromagnetic interference that the electrical system generates is biologically harmful to the human.

Regarding the transmitting gas meters, I saw South West Gas take the manual meter reading at my home in December 2013 while I was out walking with my partner and our baby. A car stopped at our home and two men got out and went into the meter area. They came out and drove off. They were stopped for about two minutes. The car had a large antenna system on the roof which I suspect is how they are currently obtaining the electronic meter readings. My community has both the old (Itron 40G) and the new style (Itron 100G) AMR/AMI gas meters. The old style appears to need to receive a signal from the car to start broadcasting, while the new type broadcasts pulsed radiation continuously. The car drove past us and we were about fifteen feet from the antenna system on its roof. I monitored our health after the AMR/AMI gas meter mobile transceiver car came through our area at lunchtime and I observed the following:

Day 1

- Skull pains that were off and on for a few hours.

- Headache appeared by 15:00 and lasted for a few hours before subsiding on its own.

- Extreme fatigue showed up at 17:00 and lasted a couple of hours. I was falling asleep while trying to have a conversation with a guest.

Day 2

- Woke up extremely thirsty.

- Headache developed during the morning that lasted all day.

- I became nauseous between 15:00 to 18:00.

- Intestinal pains in the evening.

- Thought patterns were off with some confusion and forgetfulness.

- Had to go to bed early due to an intolerable headache.

- Insomnia through the night.

- My three month old baby woke up two hours earlier than normal, was fussy, restless and refused to sleep more than half an hour at a time. Her behaviors were distinctly different from her usual routine of sleeping for a couple of hours between feeds.

- Baby spitting up far more than usual.

Day 3

- My partner had to look after the baby as I had become so sick.

- Got out of bed at 12:00 with a severe headache that lasted all day.

- Hearing in both ears was showing issues that lasted all day. The sensitivity kept on changing.

- Baby woke up 2 hours earlier than normal.

- Baby spitting up far more than usual.

Day 4

- Headache all day long.

- Baby woke up 2 hours earlier than normal.

- Baby spitting up far more than usual.

Day 5

- Skull pains came back and were infrequent during the day.

- My partner was showing the Neurasthenia symptom of irritability.

- Baby woke up 2 hours earlier than normal.

- Baby screamed in pain for two hours and was inconsolable.

Day 6, 7 and 8

- Skull pains came back and were infrequent during the day.

The above appeared to be the biological reaction to the spike in radiation levels that occurred as all of the AMR transmitting meters in the area started to broadcast their radiation and to the gas company car radio frequency transmitter. I am wondering what radiation is being broadcast from that meter reading car to see such a severe set of reactions. I have not seen such a diverse and severe sickness for quite some time, so it was an unusual event for me. It may not have occurred had I been sitting inside the home as opposed to outside walking with the baby where the man-made radiation levels are much higher. I would suggest that if you see the utility meter reading car in your area, that you should probably go indoors for the rest of the day in order to protect your health.

I am sure that you would agree that these are concerning effects from the simple action of having gas meters read by the gas company! My partner had the same exposures and showed much milder effects as she is about three times less sensitive to radiation exposures than I am. She does not have any metal dental bridges that act as an antenna system that I have. I am very concerned that my three month old daughter had this exposure to her ovaries and this may have an impact on her fertility later in life. We will find out in about four decades from now what her lasting effects are to this exposure. This was clearly a case of electronic assault by the gas utility company on my family.

The Tucson utilities Itron AMR/AMI radiation transmitting metering system is by far the most toxic transmitting system that I have come across in three years of biological radio frequency research. It is orders of magnitude more toxic than anything else that I have encountered. I have walked right up to the forest of high powered transmitters in the antenna park on Sandia Peak in Alberqueque, New Mexico, and have not seen reactions anything like this. The radiation levels are so high next to that antenna park that there are posted warnings in the car

park! It is likely that many people are adversely reacting to the utility transmitting meter reading car and have not yet associated their sickness that occurs to the biologically harmful exposure. They are likely getting approximately a week of sickness every time it passes through their neighborhood.

It is clear from the many plant growth experiments that I have performed with the Dieffenbachia plant that an atmospheric DC voltage has gone missing in the modern world and this lack of DC atmospheric voltage is having far reaching consequences for all life where it is not present. It appears that a great biological price has been paid by the modern masses for the convenience of tall man-made structures, electricity and wireless radiation.

Today I have health that I thought impossible to achieve just a few months ago in this home. While I have been able to alleviate some of the symptoms that showed up when the Itron 100G transmitting gas meter was installed throughout my community, the symptom of occasional daytime fatigue is proving difficult to shake off and is in line with living in an unnaturally high radio frequency field. The biological toxins that I am being exposed to concern me. It is well known in the electromagnetic community that people who are showing mild symptoms of electromagnetic stress typically have blood composition that matches the people who are showing severe stress. The blood composition tends to be abnormal either way!

It appears that I have now reached the point where I have to move home. There are simply too many environmental problems that I cannot rectify at my home. My impression from dealing with the utilities and government regulators is that my home is simply typical of the average American home! This also matches my assessment of homes that I have performed measurements in around the Tucson area. The problems at my home appear to be quite mild when compared to others that I have visited in the Tucson area. I find this very concerning. There comes a point where you have to acknowledge that some environmental variables are outside of your control and you have to move to rectify them. These are:

- Stray voltage/current/frequency on my tiled flooring, toilets, baths and showers from the electrical utility system in the street. (Electrical utility and Arizona Corporation Commission refuses to fix it, even though it is deforming my garden plants at the front of the home and houseplants inside the home).

- Neighbors wireless radiation emissions including their transmitting utility meters. (Gas utility, Arizona Corporation Commission and the Federal Communications Commission refuses to remove the neighbor's Itron 100G AMR gas meter that is just 15 feet from my home, even though I have a doctors letter stating that I should not be exposed to these radiation emissions).

- The radio frequency radiation environment of Tucson, Arizona, is heavily overloaded by many forms of wireless communication systems. The town appears to have radio frequency levels that averages around 1,000 mV/m and peaks to over 2,000 mV/m at homes and businesses that I have measured. (The Tenmars TM-196 RF meter states "*We recommend a maximum level of 614 mV/m for prolonged exposure*")

- Sonic boom infra-sound waves passing through my area. (The military bombing range is not moving any time soon).

The utilities and corporate governments are fully aware that they are making many people in their own populations sick. They are completely okay with this. Your sickness is nothing more than an "Inconvenient Truth" to their profit making empires that they have created. The causes of human sickness will be willfully ignored while massive profits are abundant. This is evidenced by the utilities not removing their toxic pulsing wireless transmitting devices from homes that have sick people in them who are unsuccessfully trying to get them removed. It

is simply a blatant violation of the basic human right to a healthy and safe life.

So how is my health today in 2014? I have definitely seen the effects that Dr. John Nash Ott talked about in his books and I have also seen them in people that I have worked with. I have had large exposures to these electromagnetic field effects for 26 years now and I am relatively healthy. I managed to recover the majority of my memory, but I do not think it will ever fully recover back to what it was prior to 2009. The exposures that I got from the high powered utility solar photovoltaic power system were extremely biologically toxic to the human mind. I do not take any medications and I eat mostly organic food and drink utility faucet water. I keep track of my daily outdoor sunlight exposure to make sure that I get sufficient daily exposure in the shade in a natural green environment. I now spend every day in rooms that have "Full Spectrum" acrylic windows. I keep my nighttime lighting low and use 120 volt soft white filament light bulbs in my home.

My health at 43 years of age is comparable to what I saw in my late teens. What I did not know in my late teens was that I was working in very high radio frequency fields at the city center hospital. I can far exceed the health that I had in my late teens by going into the countryside where I obtain near perfect health.

In 2009 the doctors could not diagnose what was wrong with me, they were telling me that I was getting old and it was a normal aspect of aging. I now know that they were misleading me, as what I had was not a normal aspect of aging. My health was at its worst in 2009 and I could only work due to taking prescription drugs. Without the drugs I would have been constantly sleeping day and night and unable to work. I no longer need any drugs of any kind and I have excellent sleep patterns. My health is 90% recovered and I can fully recover it by going into rural areas that have little pollution. I do have to conclude at this point that the reason why I cannot get 100% health at my home is due to incorrect human environmental conditions.

This matches the growth patterns that I observe in the Dieffenbachia (Dumb Cane) plants. After two years of growing these at my home, I can only get them to show improved growth patterns that are similar to the original growth by connecting them to 1.5 volt batteries, grounding the pot to the closest tiled floor to my back garden, putting a battery powered resin strap wrist watch with a second hand in the roots, and watering with tea. Without this type of intervention, they show excessive deformity.

Based on what I see with these plants, I have to conclude that modern cities and suburban areas have a level of biological toxicity associated with them. This toxicity is increasing with each year of the wireless revolution. This matches what we are seeing in the children. Autism is an accelerating disease in the children and there are no doubts today that electromagnetic interference exposures are driving it. The children are like the canaries in the cage, when they are not developing properly, you know you have got some really serious human environmental problems!

I think that 90% of full health is the best that a person can obtain in a suburban environment. I think that it may be even lower in a city environment due to the wireless radiation overloading and "Full City Health" may only be at 80%. The only way a person can obtain 100% health in a wireless radiation society is to go to rural areas. I do believe that I have obtained at this point what I call "Full Suburban Health". I do prefer what I call "Full Rural Health" and my future plans revolve around moving to a rural area that has little wireless radiation pollution. Unfortunately, such areas are rapidly disappearing and there is no escaping satellite transmissions.

I do consider Tucson, Arizona, to be a biologically toxic town as many properties have three AMR radiation transmitting utility meters on them. Add in the sonic boom infra-sound emissions, the high radio frequency levels and the stray voltage problems from the dry desert electrical grounding systems and it is a really toxic mess! If you are considering moving to Tucson, I would recommend that you go to a different town that does not have these biological problems. Tucson has a high rate of Autism that is likely related to these problems.

Remote National Parks offer the ability to assess if your health symptoms are being caused by electrical exposures, transmitter systems and window glazing in your environment. Most transmitter systems are banned from National Parks and that includes cell phone towers. So take a camping trip and engage in outdoor activities for a few weeks and see if your health improves there. Be careful though, as you may initially go into withdrawal! The withdrawal will be similar to cold and flu symptoms and should clear up after a week or so.

There is only one reason why I am relatively healthy today and that is because I detoxified from the radiation exposures after discovering that I had radiation sickness.

So, as you can see, I have had quite a journey through the realms of human health issues. My conclusion is that the majority of ailments that humans suffer from are caused by incorrect environmental exposures. Both sunlight and electrical systems are sources of radiation exposures and you need to be aware of your exposure to these.

You should spend time characterizing your body and establish the correct daily level of outdoor sunlight exposure for it. You should also characterize your electrical environment and reduce your exposures as much as possible to electrical systems and products. You should only have the exposures that are absolutely necessary in order to do what you need to do. The more exposures you have to electricity then the more likely it is to impact your health. These health effects appear in most people as general poor health and compromised mental functioning.

Regarding children, you should avoid purchasing electrical, electronic and wireless toys for them. It is preferable to also turn off the electrical circuit in their bedroom. Developing children should not be sleeping in rooms that have electricity in them. Do not purchase a television or laptop computer for their rooms, as the electromagnetic fields are too large for their developing cells to cope with in the long term. With developing children you should be keeping their environment as natural as possible.

It is preferable to arrange your rooms and use common sense so that you are not exposed to easily avoidable electromagnetic fields. Some simple steps are:

- Do not walk barefoot on conductive flooring that has stray voltage on it.

- Do not urinate into toilets that have stray voltage on the water.

- Keep chairs away from walls.

- Avoid putting chairs within 10 feet of a television in all directions.

- Be aware of what products are on the other side of the walls.

- Do not put chairs near to large appliances like cookers, microwave ovens, refrigerators, washers, and dryers.

- Stay away from electrical fuse boards and utility meters.

- Be aware of what is under the floor on upper story's and avoid the electromagnetic hotspots that may appear in the floor.

- Use wooden furniture.

- Sleep on a natural foam mattress on a low wooden bed frame far away from the electrical fuse board and utility transmitting meters.

- Your bedroom should be free of electricity and electrical, electronic and wireless products.

- Do not use radioactive ionizing smoke detectors, have optical ones instead.

- Do not use wireless products.

- Use only the electrical and electronic products that you need. Unplug them when not in use.

- Use filament light bulbs.

- Be aware of the transmitters in your local neighborhood.
- Pay attention to the locations of streetlights and power poles near your home.

Good health for most people is easy to achieve and it just takes some simple adjustments in lifestyle. The adjustments are far easier than expensive visits to the doctor and mentally challenged children.

"The only people mad at you for speaking the TRUTH are those living a lie. Keep speaking it."

Unknown

Summary

The value of nature to humanity is infinite. There has been a lack of understanding of the functions that nature provides to humanity that is clearly instinctively present in young children and native people. This lack of understanding has led to widespread illness, disease, cancer, and mental health issues in the modern population.

The destruction and detachment from the natural environment that the modern human has displayed will be regarded as one of the biggest mistakes ever made in human history. The pollution of the atmosphere, rivers and oceans is already acknowledged as an environmental catastrophe that has led to the extinction of millions of species.

It is common to see headlines that underline the failing modern society, such as *"Diabetes Rate Doubles"* or *"UK Depression Rate Up by 40%"*. Diabetes and depression are modern diseases born out of the Industrial Revolution, as are so many of the modern diseases. It is quite a simple progression to where we are today:

- Cutting the trees down significantly increased the ground based radiation levels that the human was exposed to. It also removed the tree canopy that has a DC voltage on it. This led to an increase in illness and disease. This appears to be the start of widespread mental illness in the human race.

- The adoption of electricity led to the regular exposure of electromagnetic interference in the human body. This corresponded to another increase in illness, disease, cancer, and mental health issues. New illnesses and diseases were born with the progression of electricity. Many babies became too large to fit through the birth canal.

- Drinking incorrect water and eating poor quality food has caused many health conditions to occur.

- Allowing the human mind and body to atrophy has opened up the human to many illnesses and diseases that were not present before the adoption of sedentary lifestyles.

- The continued pollution of the atmosphere, rivers, and oceans is increasing human illness, disease, cancer, and mental health issues, and the continuation of this process should be expected to lead to human extinction.

Illness, disease, cancer, mental health issues and altered growth rates in babies and children are the current fruits of modern society. There is no mystery about cancer, it is the disease of pollution. Unfortunately, when it comes to pollution and human health, cancer is just the tip of the iceberg. Without the environment, we are all dead.

I have every expectation that in the future, electricity will be regarded in the same way that asbestos and smoking are viewed today. The electrification of the ground that we walk on can only be described as the actions of an insane race of people. Stray voltage effects, biological field coupling, toxic artificial lighting products and willingly electrifying the air with radio and microwaves will be documented by future historians as the peak of human insanity. Indeed, the historical records indicate that Nikola Tesla, the inventor of many of the modern systems that we routinely use, may have been one of the earliest documented cases of environmental and electromagnetic hypersensitivity!

The most polluted animal on the planet today is the modern human.

It is time to change back to a nature based society and put the Industrial Revolution behind us as an unfortunate mistake in human history. Never again should we have nations whose measure of success is how much money they can make. Rather, nations should be using nature based standards to gauge their success. There should be no higher standard than the health and well-being of their children and their elderly people.

Nature is well documented as bringing about positive health and mental well being. Research findings include:

- Better cognitive functioning.
- More self discipline and impulse control.
- Greater overall mental health.
- Enhanced recovery from surgery.
- Enable and support higher levels of physical activity.
- Improved immune system functioning.
- Improved memory.

Less access to nature is linked to:

- Exacerbated attention deficit/hyperactivity disorder symptoms.
- Higher rates of anxiety disorders.
- Higher rates of clinical depression.
- Greater rates of childhood obesity.
- Higher rates of overall disease.
- Higher rates of mortality in younger and older adults.

Here is what appears to be the recipe for good human health:

- Drinking hot tea made with hard mineralized water.
- Fresh air in a natural outdoor environment.

- Fresh organic food of mainly fruits and vegetables.

- Daily high activity strength exercises.

- No industrial sound or vibration waves.

- An outdoor solar radiation environment that is modified by the tree canopy.

- An annual hibernation cycle.

- Correct daily exposure to solar radiation.

- Exposure to the natural DC atmospheric voltage.

- No unnatural electromagnetic interference (EMI) effects.

- No man-made chemicals.

- A supportive social structure that recognizes and promotes the beneficial effects that nature is providing to the human mind and body.

Energy fields define who we are as humans. If you are in environments that are creating positive energy, then you will have excellent mental and physical health. If you are in environments where the energy levels are negative, then you will fall into poor mental and physical health. Unfortunately, today's modern society has created far more negative energy fields and finding good mental and physical health is becoming increasingly difficult.

Feng Shui is the study of positive energy in the human environment. It literally means wind and water. The people who developed Feng Shui understood that human emotions and health were governed by their environments. If you are feeling ill or having emotional issues, you should apply the science of Feng Shui to your environment as it will probably help a lot. You cannot go wrong by having an environment that has the science of Feng Shui applied to it.

I never thought that I would be using my Red Cross and St. Johns medical training, biomedical background, astronomical skills and my electrical & electronic engineering degree that I obtained in my twenties to fix the health problems that showed up in my thirties. My skills turned out to be very useful, far more effective than any doctor I saw. I do find it rather strange that to live in modern society that I have to behave like I am on the International Space Station! This lifestyle underscores how alien the modern human environment has become.

The book "Harmony" by the Prince of Wales has provided an excellent road map back to where we need to be. Harmony with nature has always been known to be the way to live a long, natural, pain-free, and healthy life.

I hope that you enjoyed the book and I wish you the very best of health.

"Every human being is the author of his own health or disease."

Sivanada

References

- Bell Hooks.
- Bill Gates.
- Clea Duvall.
- Deepak Chopra.
- Do Trees Strengthen Urban Communities, Reduce Domestic Violence? Paper by By W. C. Sullivan, Ph.D. & Frances E. Kuo, Ph.D.
- Dr. George Crile.
- Dr. Jim Burch: http://cpcp.sph.sc.edu/fs/burch.htm
- Dr. John Nash Ott:

  http://www.biolightgroup.com/Ott.html
- Dr. Magda Havas: http://www.magdahavas.com/
- Dr. Philip Stoddard: http://www2.fiu.edu/~stoddard/
- Dr. Samuel Milham MD MPH: http://www.sammilham.com/
- Dr. William Rae: http://www.ecopolitan.com/dr-william-rae
- Earthing: The Most Important Health Discovery Ever? by Clinton Ober, Stephen T. Sinatra and Martin Zucker: http://earthinginstitute.net/
- Edward Stanley.
- Electrocution of America: Is Your Utility Company Out to Kill You? by Russ Allen.
- Elizabeth Kelley MA, Director of the Electromagnetic Safety Alliance.
- Eric Schmidt.
- Francis Bacon.

- Frank Lloyd Wright.

- Frederick Douglass.

- Freeman Dyson.

- Galileo Galilei.

- Google Maps: http://maps.google.com

- Henry Beston.

- Henry St. John.

- John F. Kennedy.

- Joyce Carol Oates.

- Leonardo da Vinci.

- Les Brown.

- Light, Radiation, and You - How to Stay Healthy by Dr. John N. Ott.

- Marilyn vos Savant.

- Martin Luther King.

- myfoxny.com article *America's anger epidemic: why?*

- Patrick Swayze.

- Plan B 4.0: Mobilizing to Save Civilization by Lester R. Brown.

- Plato.

- Popular Science: http://www.popsci.com/science/article/2010-02/disconnected

- Sivanada.

- Stetzer Electric: http://www.stetzerelectric.com/

- Ted Scambos.

- Tom Stoppard.

- UNC Terrorism Research:
  http://www.unc.edu/spotlight/terrorism_research
- Virginia Woolf.
- William Wordsworth.
- Wikipedia: http://www.wikipedia.org/

"None of us is as smart as all of us."
Eric Schmidt

Internet

Manufacturers of ultraviolet (UV) transmitting full spectrum acrylic window glazing sheets are:

Lucite International, Inc: LuciteLux UTRAN UVT:
http://www.lucitelux.com/product.aspx?productID=4

Spartech: Solacryl "Monkey-Shine" SUVT:
http://www.spartech.com/polycast/Spartech-Polycast-Solacryl-Monkey-Shine.pdf

Vitamin D Wiki is a useful collection of vitamin D information:
http://vitamindwiki.com/VitaminDWiki

Useful electromagnetic websites are:

Bioinitiative Report is a rationale for biologically-based public exposure standards for electromagnetic fields (ELF and RF):
http://www.bioinitiative.org/

Dr. Magda Havas, PhD, co-author of "Public Health SOS: The Shadow Side of the Wireless Revolution":
http://www.magdahavas.com/

Dr. Nina Pierpont is developing the health effects of wind turbines and infrasound: http://www.windturbinesyndrome.com/

Dr. Samuel Milham, author of "Dirty Electricity":

http://www.sammilham.com/

ElectroSensitivity UK is a website that aims to provide unbiased and balanced information to help those who have become sensitive to mobile and cordless phones, their masts, WiFi, and a multitude of common everyday electrical appliances: http://www.es-uk.info/

Environmental Health Center-Dallas, Texas, medically tests and treats human health problems including sensitivities to pollens, molds, dust, foods, chemicals, air (indoor/outdoor), water, electromagnetic sensitivity (EMF), and many more health problems as they relate to our environment: http://www.ehcd.com/

Environmental Radiation LLC offers the services to identify the modern invisible toxins that we are routinely exposed to and the know-how to rectify the problems.

http://www.environmentalradiation.com/

FEB - The Swedish Association for the ElectroHyperSensitive:

http://www.feb.se/index_int.htm

Guidelines of the Austrian Medical Association for the diagnosis and treatment of EMF related health problems and illnesses (EMF syndrome)

http://freiburger-appell-2012.info/media/EMF%20Guideline %20OAK-AG%20%202012%2003%2003.pdf

Less EMF are a leading supplier in the USA of electromagnetic radiation products: http://www.lessemf.com/

Mast-Victims.org - An international community website for people suffering adverse health effects from mobile phone masts in the vicinity of their homes

http://www.mast-victims.org/

Medical Perspective on Environmental Sensitivities - Canadian Human Rights Commission: http://www.chrc-ccdp.gc.ca/sites/default/files/envsensitivity_en.pdf

Powerwatch UK: http://www.powerwatch.org.uk/

Smart Meter Opposition Groups in the United States of America:

http://www.takebackyourpower.net/directory/us/

Stetzer Electric, Inc, manufacturers of the STETZERiZER® Filter:

http://www.stetzerelectric.com/

WEEP - The Canadian initiative to stop wireless, electric, and electromagnetic pollution: http://www.weepinitiative.org/

World Health Organization (WHO) International Workshop on Electromagnetic Field Hypersensitivity: http://www.who.int/peh-emf/publications/reports/EHS_Proceedings_June2006.pdf

"The Internet is becoming the town square for the global village of tomorrow."

Bill Gates

Acknowledgments

This book was influenced by:

- My father for his discussions about how the fat content in meat changes color between diary cows and open range cows.

- Claudia Sandoval M.S.W. for her wisdom on trees and how it relates in the social environment.

- My neighbors for their understanding and assistance with my biological experiments.

- Dr. John Nash Ott for his extensive research into health, light, and radiation. His lasting legacy of publications was a wonderful gift to the next generation:

  - My Ivory Cellar; [the story of time-lapse photography].

  - Health and Light: The Extraordinary Study That Shows How Light Affects Your Health and Emotional Well Being.

  - Light, Radiation, and You: How to Stay Healthy.

  - Color and Light: Their Effects on Plants, Animals and People.

  - Exploring the Spectrum: The Effects of Natural and Artificial Light on Living Organisms.

- The numerous people and companies who are referenced in this book that have worked diligently to bring the important science of environmental health to the masses.

"Help others achieve their dreams and you will achieve yours."
Les Brown

About the Author

Steven started his career at one of the largest university research and teaching hospitals in Europe. Working in the electrical engineering group, he obtained a Bachelors with Honors in Electrical and Electronic Engineering. Human health was a strong draw and he moved into the biomedical team, serving the regions hospitals. During this time he developed a fascination for human illness and disease and the causes of it, many of which were not understood.

He joined the Isaac Newton Group of Telescopes in 1999 and went to live in La Palma. La Palma is part of the Canary Islands, governed by Spain. During this time he worked with the leading European astronomers and developed his astronomical and optics skills. He became fluent in Spanish and their culture.

In 2001 he became a Chartered Electrical Engineer and joined the W. M. Keck Observatory in Hawaii. This was the world's leading astronomical facility and home to the world's two largest segmented mirror telescopes. Steven developed segmented optics and interferometry skills while working alongside world leading astronomers. During this time Steven constructed his own off-grid solar powered home in the last of the traditional Hawaiian fishing villages in Miloli'i, Hawaii. He learned Hawaiian Pidgin English and the Hawaiian culture during his time there.

In 2006, Steven became the Director of the MDM Observatory in Sells, Arizona, USA. Working for Columbia University and later, Dartmouth College, he developed the facility to modern standards. He learned an appreciation of the native Americans and their culture from the Tohono O'odham Nation.

In 2008, Steven joined the solar power revolution that was sweeping the USA and commissioned the largest CIGS thin film solar photovoltaic installation in the world.

A year later he commissioned the largest solar photovoltaic power plant in the USA. The system rated power was quoted as 25,000,000 watts AC with over 90,500 solar modules that were mounted to 158 single-axis tracker systems in three hundred acres of land.

He went on to develop the solar photovoltaic team for a large international company.

In 2010 he started to research radiation and publish the leading books on the subject.

"All truths are easy to understand once they are discovered; the point is to discover them."

Galileo Galilei

Author Contact

I hope that you found the book informative and please let me know about any questions or comments about the book. I can be contacted through the StevenMageeBooks channel on www.youtube.com.

I am a consultant in the areas that I research at Environmental Radiation LLC and please feel free to contact me for any help or assistance. This is the website:

http://www.environmentalradiation.com/

You can follow the twitter feed at:

Steven Magee @EnvironmentEMR

The Facebook page is:

https://www.facebook.com/EnvironmentEMR

You may find my other books useful:

Solar Photovoltaic

- **Complete Solar Photovoltaics for Residential, Commercial, and Utility Systems:** Steven Magee has combined his three top selling books on solar power systems into one edition. Complete Solar Photovoltaics will train you on solar photovoltaics and show you how to design grid connected solar photovoltaic power systems. Operations and maintenance is detailed to enable you to have a complete understanding of solar photovoltaics from start to finish.

- **Solar Photovoltaics for Consumers, Utilities, and Investors:** This book details solar photovoltaic systems for consumers, utilities and investors. This would encompass residential, commercial and utility systems that are connected to the utility grid. There is a discussion of the different technologies available for the consumer and their advantages and disadvantages. For the utilities, there is invaluable advice on planning and constructing large projects. For the investor, forward looking statements try to predict the future of solar photovoltaics.

- **Solar Photovoltaic Training for Residential, Commercial, and Utility Systems:** This book details solar photovoltaic training for those who are interested in this area and also for those who are already working in the field. This would encompass residential, commercial, and utility systems that are connected to the utility grid. It is a comprehensive overview of a rapidly growing world of solar photovoltaic power generation technology.

- **Solar Photovoltaic Design for Residential, Commercial, and Utility Systems:** This book details how to design reliable solar photovoltaic power generation systems from a residential system, progressing to a commercial system, and finishing at the largest utility power generation systems. By following the guidelines in this book and your local solar photovoltaic electrical codes, you will be able to design trouble free solar power systems that give many years of reliable operation. When designed well, solar photovoltaic power generation is an excellent source of electrical power that results in much lower electricity bills, the power company will even refund you for the excess energy generated by your system if it is large enough. Building a grid tied solar power system is a relatively easy task. Given the large amount of government and electrical utility financial incentives that are available, it is a great time to join in the solar power revolution that is taking place in the world today.

- **Solar Photovoltaic Operation and Maintenance for Residential, Commercial, and Utility Systems:** This book details how to operate and maintain residential, commercial, and utility solar photovoltaic systems that are connected to the utility grid. By following the guidelines in this book you will be able to operate and maintain solar power systems that should give many years of reliable operation. Invaluable trouble shooting advice will aid in returning your system to full operation in the event of a problem.

- **Solar Photovoltaic DC Calculations for Residential, Commercial, and Utility Systems:** This book details how to run calculations for the DC circuit of solar photovoltaic systems. This would encompass residential, commercial, and utility systems that are connected to the utility grid. It covers the range of conditions that solar photovoltaic modules are exposed to throughout the year and shows how to incorporate these into an effective DC circuit that is well designed and reliable.

- **Solar Photovoltaic Resource for Residential, Commercial, and Utility Systems:** This book is a resource of information that is used in the solar photovoltaic field. This would encompass residential, commercial, and utility systems that are connected to the utility grid. It is a comprehensive collection of notes, diagrams, pictures and charts for a rapidly growing world of solar photovoltaic power generation technology. This book is illustrated in color.

Solar

- **Solar Irradiance and Insolation for Power Systems:** This book is a resource of information that is used in the solar power generation field. This would encompass residential, commercial, and utility systems that are connected to the utility grid. It is a comprehensive collection of notes, diagrams, pictures, and charts for a rapidly growing world of solar photovoltaic power generation technology. This book is illustrated in color.

- **Solar Site Selection for Power Systems:** This book is a comprehensive collection of images, diagrams, and notes that document the effects of light and heat in the solar power generation field. This would encompass residential, commercial, and utility systems that are connected to the utility grid. This is essential information for a rapidly growing world of solar power generation technology. This book is illustrated in color.

Architecture

- **Solar Reflections for Architects, Engineers, and Human Health:** This book is a comprehensive collection of images, diagrams, and notes that document the effects of sunlight in architecture. This is essential information for architects, engineers, and the medical profession. The discovery of the "Multiple-Sun" effect in architecture is detailed and this book is illustrated in color.

Human Health

- **Solar Radiation – A Cause of Illness and Cancer?** Illness and cancers have become part of our modern culture. It has been discovered that extremely high levels of man-made solar radiation exist in modern society. Could this be the one of the causes of illness and cancers? This book examines the increase in solar radiation and applies it to human health.

- **Solar Radiation, Global Warming, and Human Disease:** This book examines the modern development of the Earth and the potential impacts on global warming and human disease. The destruction of the forests for modern agricultural use appears to have effects that are not fully understood and these are explored. Radiation deficiency and radiation overloading are investigated to see if they are factors in many illnesses and diseases.

- **Toxic Light:** Toxic Light takes a look at the light pollution that may be in your local environment and relates it to the health problems that it may cause. Light in the human environment is only just starting to be understood and something as innocent as your sunglasses may be able to make you ill! There are many examples of commonplace items in your environment that may have the ability to affect your health. Get ready for enlightenment about the most important human nutrient of light!

- **Toxic Health:** Toxic Health takes a look at the pollution that may be in your local environment and relates it to the health problems that it can cause. Pollution in the human environment is only just starting to be understood and something as innocent as light may be able to make you really ill! There are many examples of commonplace items in your environment that may have the ability to affect your health. In particular, we will investigate if modern city life is the most toxic thing of all to the modern human!

- **Toxic Electricity:** Random aches and pains? Fatigue? Insomnia? Facial pains? Irregular heartbeats? Sick kids? Relationship problems? Blotchy skin? Anxiety? Toxic electricity takes a look at the electrical system and asks the question: Is this one of the most toxic endeavors that humanity has ever engaged in?

Forensics

- **Electrical Forensics:** Electrical Forensics examines the many aspects of electricity, electronics and wireless communications that may lead to unusual behaviors to occur in humans. Electromagnetic interference is well known for its ability to affect mental functioning and human health. Electrical Forensics demonstrates how to identify toxic electromagnetic environments that may be the root cause of accidents and crimes.

- **Health Forensics:** Health Forensics examines the many aspects of modern society that may lead to unusual behaviors to occur in humans. Modern society has adopted habits that are well known for their ability to affect mental functioning and human health. Health Forensics demonstrates how to identify toxic human environments that may be the root cause of accidents and crimes.

Religion

- **Solar Radiation, the Book of Revelations, and the Era of Light – Part 1:** Welcome to the Era of Light! Light has long been known to be essential nourishment for the human body. We will explore the different types of light that are present on Earth and relate it to human health and nature. Light is discussed extensively in the Bible and we will see if we can associate our findings to it. Finally, we will investigate if the Industrial Revolution has created the ultimate toxin of poisonous sunlight!

Professional

- **Engineering Science and Education Journal Volume: 11, Issue: 4, Active Control Systems for Large Segmented Optical Mirrors:** A new generation of optical telescopes is on the drawing board. These will be true giants with primary mirrors having a diameter of up to 100 meters. The technology that will enable this revolution to take place was developed at the W. M. Keck Observatory in Hawaii, where the world's largest segmented mirrors are in daily use. This article looks at how the W. M. Keck Observatory proved the mirror technology that will be behind this new generation of telescopes.

You can search "Steven Magee Books" for the very latest publications.

www.youtube.com videos supporting the ideas in the books can be found by searching: StevenMageeBooks

"Life-transforming ideas have always come to me through books."

Bell Hooks

Book Reviews

Electrical Forensics rated 5 out of 5 stars.

Review by John Puccetti on October 27, 2013 titled "Dangers of electricity"

Steven has made many of the health problems of our century known in his book. But what will we do is this information? We live in a corporate dictatorship that masquerades as democracy.

Toxic Electricity rated 5 out of 5 stars.

Review by Sam Wieder on December 13, 2013 titled "A Most Illuminating, Educational, and Helpful Book"

Toxic Electricity provides a clear and comprehensive description of the many ways in which electrical fields impact human health and offers simple steps that anyone can take to live a more vibrant life in our electrically toxic world. The author does a masterful job of presenting some fairly complex concepts in a way that is easily understandable. Reading this book will give you a deeper understanding of how unseen radiation in your living and working environment may be impacting you. If you've been battling different health challenges or are chronically tired for no apparent reason, this book may very well open your eyes to some answers that will help you regain your health and your life.

Peter Sullivan @petermsullivan9 twittered on 10th December 2013:

@EnvironmentEMR Thanks for writing about the #autism / #EMF theory in you book Toxic Electricity. Also love the use of plants as "canaries".

Toxic Electricity: Eric Van rated it 5 out of 5 stars on Dec 23, 2012

If you think that you're home or work environment is safe and sound think again. If you are fatigued or have strange ailments currently or are concerned about cancer in the future then I recommend reading this book and getting an education into how you can avoid the toxins you receive from electricity.

Toxic Light rated 4 out of 5 Stars.

Review by John Puccetti on January 2, 2014 titled "Very technical".

I recommend you read "Tesla a man out of time" before you read this book. It is hard to grasp how much is wrong with radio frequencies and the electric grid and smart meters unless you really do some research first. But it is a wake up call to us all. Well worth reading.

"A good, sympathetic review is always a wonderful surprise."

Joyce Carol Oates